WAIST DISPOSAL

THE ULTIMATE
FAT LOSS
MANUAL FOR MEN

Dr John Briffa

HAY HOUSE

HAY HOUSE
Australia • Canada • Hong Kong • India
South Africa • United Kingdom • United States

First published and distributed in the United Kingdom by:

Hay House UK Ltd, 292B Kensal Rd, London W10 5BE. Tel.: (44) 20 8962 1230; Fax: (44) 20 8962 1239. www.hayhouse.co.uk

Published and distributed in the United States of America by:

Hay House, Inc., PO Box 5100, Carlsbad, CA 92018-5100. Tel.: (1) 760 431 7695 or (800) 654 5126; Fax: (1) 760 431 6948 or (800) 650 5115. www.hayhouse.com

Published and distributed in Australia by:

Hay House Australia Ltd, 18/36 Ralph St, Alexandria NSW 2015. Tel.: (61) 2 9669 4299; Fax: (61) 2 9669 4144. www.hayhouse.com.au

Published and distributed in the Republic of South Africa by:

Hay House SA (Pty), Ltd, PO Box 990, Witkoppen 2068. Tel./Fax: (27) 11 467 8904. www.hayhouse.co.za

Published and distributed in India by:

Hay House Publishers India, Muskaan Complex, Plot No.3, B-2, Vasant Kunj, New Delhi – 110 070. Tel.: (91) 11 4176 1620; Fax: (91) 11 4176 1630. www.hayhouse.co.in

Distributed in Canada by:

Raincoast, 9050 Shaughnessy St, Vancouver, BC V6P 6E5. Tel.: (1) 604 323 7100; Fax: (1) 604 323 2600

© Dr John Briffa, 2010

DISCLAIMER: The information contained in this book is not intended as a replacement for professional medical advice. Any use of the information in this book is at the reader's discretion. The author and the publisher specifically disclaim any and all liability arising directly or indirectly from the use or application of any information contained in this book. A healthcare professional should be consulted regarding your specific health situation and before you start a new exercise regime.

A catalogue record for this book is available from the British Library.

ISBN 978-1-84850-115-7.

Printed in the UK by CPI William Clowes Beccles NR34 7TL

CONTENTS

INTRODUCTION

Let's cut to the chase: The fact that you've picked up this book means, in all likelihood, that you're carrying a bit of a belly that you'd rather be rid of. Maybe you're a bit frustrated that despite spurts of healthy eating and get fit campaigns over the years, your weight has been on an unrelenting upward trend. Do you sometimes find yourself lamenting the fact that clothes that once fitted perfectly are now languishing in a wardrobe or drawer because you can no longer get into them? Maybe you've seen your doctor recently and have been warned that your weight is posing a risk to your health and wellbeing. Irrespective of the nature of your weight issue and whatever your goal, *Waist Disposal* is here to help.

In this book you will find comprehensive, practical and easy-to-apply information and advice designed for effective, permanent fat loss. An improved, more athletic physique can be yours, too. And all you need to transform your body for the better is to follow some simple dietary guidelines that have nothing to do with calorie counting or portion control (so no hunger), and exercise for just 12 minutes a day.

How can I be so sure that the information here works? Because, as a practising doctor specialising in nutritional medicine, I have spent over a decade and a half advising literally thousands of individuals on how to manage all aspects of their health, including their weight. This experience 'on the ground' has allowed me to see at first hand what works (as well as what *doesn't*) for shedding fat and enjoying significant improvements in other measures of health. The information contained in these pages is a distillate of my experiences with countless individuals who have achieved their health goals. They've done it, and you can, too.

It would not be true to claim, though, that the information and advice offered here is purely based on my clinical experience. The fact is, it is science-based, too. In this book I refer to literally hundreds of scientific studies that reveal the true causes of excess weight, as well as the most effective remedies for it (the little numbers that appear in the text refer to specific studies that are listed towards the back of the book). There is a huge mound of evidence that demonstrates the most effective ways to shed fat and enjoy long-lasting health and vitality, so why not use it?

It is this science that shows how many nutritional concepts taken as 'fact' turn out not to be true at all. For example, in this book you'll learn how, when it comes to successful weight loss, just consuming fewer calories or burning more through exercise is very rarely effective. Other myths put to bed here include the notion that fat is inherently fattening, that animal fat causes heart disease, and that artificial sweeteners aid weight loss. You'll also learn what science shows are the true causes of obesity and ill-health, and how to protect yourself from them.

You may wonder as you read this book how and why the truth about how best to optimise our weight and health runs counter to conventional wisdom. One explanation is that inaccurate information can easily be passed through the ages if it is repeated often enough and the facts aren't checked. And there's always the possibility that certain commercial concerns (e.g. elements within the food industry) will perpetuate myths because it makes good commercial sense to do so. Using up-to-date research, *Waist Disposal* dispels these myths, and separates science fact from science fiction.

Waist Disposal dishes up a healthy dose of common sense, too. Leaving the science aside for one moment, logic dictates that the best diet for us as a species is one based on the foods that we've been eating longest in terms of our time on this planet. Why? Because those are the foods we're best adapted to through the process of evolution, and are therefore most likely to meet our nutritional, metabolic and physiological needs.

Evolutionists estimate that we've been on this planet nearly 2.5 million years. For the vast majority of our time here we have been 'hunter-gatherers', subsisting on a diet made up of what might be termed 'primal' foods such as meat, fish, eggs, fruits, vegetables, nuts and seeds. Only relatively recently (about 10,000 years ago) did we start to settle in communities to grow crops of grains such as wheat and corn. Condense the whole of human evolution into a year, and it turns out we started eating grains just a day and a half ago.

Evolution is a slow, creeping process and, genetically speaking, we are virtually identical to our ancestors from 10,000 years ago. What this means is that, on the most fundamental of levels – our genetic code – the diet we are best adapted to is the diet we ate *prior* to the introduction of grain. Other nutritional 'newcomers' we might view with suspicion include refined sugar, milk and vegetable oils. As you'll see, the idea of eating a 'primal' diet is not merely a theory, but something that is supported by abundant scientific evidence.

In addition to presenting the relevant science, this book will also sometimes refer to what I term 'The Primal Principle'. Here, we will marry our ancient nutritional heritage with what science tells us about the appropriateness of specific foodstuffs. Even if you forget most (or even all!) of the scientific detail in this book, simply seeing food from an evolutionary perspective will allow you to make quick, easy and accurate decisions about the very best foods to eat.

The benefits of following the advice in this book can be profound. First and foremost, it can allow you to enjoy lasting, satisfying fat loss, including from around your midriff. This is not just important from an aesthetic standpoint. As you will discover in the first chapter (Toxic Waist), 'abdominal fat' has strong links with conditions such as heart disease and diabetes, and appears to speed our way to an early demise, too. The happy reality is that a shrinking waistline can translate into a diminishing risk of disease and premature death.

The fact that we men are prone to accumulating this most toxic form of fat is unfortunate, but there's good news for us, too. My experience in practice is that when men apply the strategies presented here, they can expect rapid results, and will generally see considerable progress within a few short weeks. This, by the way, contrasts somewhat with the generally less impressive fat losses experienced by women. One reason for this may be that men are less prone to sluggishness of the metabolism caused by, say, low thyroid function or repeated cycles of strict dieting. Whatever the explanation, the fact remains that while abdominal fat is both unsightly and unhealthy, it is something that men can almost always rid themselves of quite quickly, and without having to go to extreme lengths or superhuman effort, either.

You may have noticed that in this brief introduction I've referred repeatedly to *fat loss*, not merely weight loss. That's because when weight is lost, it's important to make sure as much of this as possible is fat, and not something more desirable like muscle. Also, if you were to lose fat and gain muscle, you might not see much change in your weight, though undoubtedly your *body composition* will have improved. The first chapter (Toxic Waist) explores this, as well as the deficiencies of the standard weight measurement – the body mass index or BMI. This chapter also offers advice on more useful measurements including waist size and body fat assessment.

The second chapter (The Calorie Trap) focuses on the calorie principle which, simply put, dictates that those who want to lose weight need to eat less or exercise more (or both). While this law has underpinned weight-loss advice for half a century, you will learn how it is dangerously flawed. You'll also discover why applying its principles so often dooms many to failure in the long term. This chapter introduces the notion that different types of food have different propensities to form fat in the body, and that when it comes to weight loss, it's more than calories that count.

After that, we get down to the business of exploring the true causes, and cures, of excess weight. Each one of the major 'macronutrients' (carbohydrate, protein and fat) will be put under the scientific spotlight. The effects that each of these has on weight and health will be explored, as will the effectiveness of different types of weight-loss diets (e.g. high-protein, low-carb, low-fat). We'll also review the published research which reveals the sort of diet that is truly the most effective for shedding unhealthy and unwanted fat. In all of this, you'll learn which foods are least likely to promote the accumulation of fat in your body.

You will also come to understand the importance of focusing your nutritional efforts on foods that are most effective at sating the appetite. This strategy is critical if we are to contain our food intake without hunger or sense of sacrifice. *Waist Disposal* reveals the most satisfying foods in our diet, as well as identifying the foodstuffs that can actually stimulate appetite and encourage overeating. So important is appetite control in successful fat loss, that I've devoted a whole chapter to it (Satisfaction Guaranteed).

But it's not all theory. *Waist Disposal* offers you a wealth of advice and information on the types of foods and meals that will assist you in your quest to banish your belly, as well as how to incorporate this dietary advice into your daily life. You'll also find recipes for tasty, easy-to-prepare meals that reflect the evidence-based nutritional principles laid out in this book. Don't worry, there's no need to be a Cordon Bleu chef – many of the recipes require very little real 'cooking', and can be knocked up in 15 minutes or less.

The nutrition information in this book is accompanied by advice regarding exercise, too. In the chapter on exercise (Muscle Bound), you'll learn that while exercise can be beneficial for a myriad of things, the rather shocking truth is that weight loss is not one of them. However, if you're serious about improving the size and strength of your musculature, then resistance exercise is a must. While this can be done in a gym, it doesn't need to be. Muscle Bound presents a daily home-based regime that can improve your muscular form in about the same time it takes to shower and shave.

While diet and exercise are cited as the two key components for weight-loss success, I suggest there is a third: our thoughts and beliefs. What goes on between our ears is a major factor in maintaining motivation for healthy habits. Plus, as you'll see, having the right mental attitude has the capacity to accelerate the benefits achieved by eating and exercising right. The final chapter (Mind Matters) offers advice on how to harness the power of your mind in order to transform your body.

Each element of *Waist Disposal* offers a truly powerful weapon for fighting flabbiness, while at the same time demanding surprisingly little in the way of effort or discipline.

No gritted-teeth determination is required here. Put the advice here to work and you can expect to be rewarded with one helluva body, but without having to go through hell to get it.

HOW TO USE THIS BOOK

If you read through this book from cover to cover, you'll perhaps recognise that the earlier chapters provide the background, much of it scientific, for the more specific and practical advice that comes later. *Waist Disposal* is written in this way because it's my belief that understanding *why* and *how* suggested changes bring about benefit helps us make and maintain those positive changes in our lives.

However, you may be an impatient sort of person, and keen to get on with things. In which case, you may want to skip a lot of theory and go to the parts of the book that are geared more to *what* to do (rather than *why* you should do it). In which case, I recommend starting at Chapter 7 (Sound Bites) and reading through to the end of the book.

However, if you do take this approach, I suggest you at least read the summaries which you will find at the end of each of the earlier chapters, under the heading 'Back to Basics'. Absorbing the key learning points here will, even without the detail, set the scene for the more practical information and advice later on. Reading these summaries may also convince you that there's enough interesting and important stuff in the earlier chapters that they're worth reading in full, even if that is at a future date.

Chapter 1

TOXIC WAIST

WHY YOUR EXPANDED WAISTLINE IS MORE THAN JUST AN EYESORE

Men and women can differ in many ways, including body shape. Differences in physique become especially pronounced when we gain weight. For men, fatty accumulation tends to be focused around the middle of the body or 'midriff'. On the other hand, women of childbearing age usually find their 'problem areas' to be the buttocks and thighs. As a result, an overweight man might be regarded as somewhat apple-like in form, while overweight women are usually more the shape of a pear.

As you'll learn in this chapter, these differences in fat distribution are not merely cosmetic. Research shows that *where* excess fat finds itself in the body influences its impact on the risk of chronic conditions such as heart disease and diabetes. And the bad news for men is that the evidence points to excess weight around the middle – known as 'abdominal obesity' – as the most toxic to health. You'll see how getting rid of your gut can have a bevy of benefits, not just in terms of how you look and feel, but for your wellness and wellbeing too.

As you apply the principles advocated in this book and see positive results, you might want to keep tabs on your progress. This chapter also reviews the usefulness of the major body measurements, starting with the most commonly used weight-related assessment of all – the body mass index or 'BMI'.

DOES THE BMI MEASURE UP?

The BMI is calculated by dividing an individual's weight in kilograms by the square of their height in metres. According to conventional wisdom, a BMI of 18.5–24.9 is regarded as 'healthy', while BMIs of 25–29.9 are considered 'overweight'. Those of 30 or above are classified as 'obese'. While the BMI usually forms the basis of the advice health professionals give to individuals about their weight, there are a number of reasons to be mistrustful of it.

First of all, the BMI tells us something about the relationship between height and weight, but nothing about *body composition*. It is entirely possible, therefore, to have a muscularly built, really very healthy individual whose BMI marks him out as 'overweight' or even 'obese'.

For example, during his playing days, rugby union back-row legend Laurence Dallaglio typically weighed in at 112 kg and stood 1.91 metres tall. Do the maths and it turns out that in his prime, Laurence Dallaglio's BMI was a shade over 30. That's right, at the top of his game our Laurence was officially *obese* (you tell him). This example demonstrates just how limited the usefulness of the BMI is in the real world.

Of course it can be that an 'obese' BMI can indeed reflect a not-so-healthy body composition. Now that Laurence Dallaglio is some way into his well-earned retirement, it's possible that his muscle mass will have dwindled, and that he may have gained some fat over time. Should this have happened, then Laurence's scale-weight and BMI may not have changed that much. A relatively static BMI may belie the fact that muscle is being lost while fat is gained. In this way, the BMI can give a false sense of security. The same, of course, is true in reverse. Someone losing fat and gaining muscle might not see much change in their weight or BMI. The bottom line is that the BMI is a fat lot of good for assessing and tracking changes in your body's *composition*.

THE BMI AS A MARKER FOR HEALTH

The fact that the BMI tells us nothing about body composition means that, in all likelihood, it's unlikely to be a good indicator of health status either. While it might be enshrined in medical lore that a 'healthy' BMI is one that ranges between 18.5 and 24.9, there is a body of evidence which suggests that is not true at all.

When considering the relationship between BMI and health, it pays to take as wide a view as possible. This is because 'lifestyle factors' such as body weight, exercise and diet can increase the risk of some conditions and reduce the risk of others. For example, drinking moderate amounts of alcohol is associated with a reduced risk of heart disease, but an increased risk of cancer. Focusing on specific medical conditions can give a skewed sense of the overall impact that any factor may have on health. Much better assessments can be made by reviewing the relationship between lifestyle factors and *overall risk of death*.

So, if BMIs of 18.5–24.9 are deemed as being the most healthy, then individuals with BMIs in this range should be at the lowest risk of dying, right? Wrong.

The biggest and most comprehensive study ever to assess the relationship between BMI and risk of death was

3

published in *Journal of the American Medical Association* in 2007.[1] Some notable findings from this study included:

- Being overweight was *not* associated with an increased risk of death from cardiovascular disease (e.g. heart attacks and strokes).

- Being overweight was *not* associated with an increased risk of death from cancer.

- Being overweight *was* associated with a *reduced* risk of death not due to cardiovascular disease or cancer.

- In individuals aged 25–59, risk of death from cardiovascular disease did not become significantly elevated until BMIs were above 35.

- There was no increased risk of death from cancer at any level of weight (even BMIs above 35).

All things considered, this study showed that being overweight might be *better* for overall survival compared to having a 'healthy' BMI. And it's not the only study that suggests that the traditional BMI categories are wide of the mark.

In a more recent study, published in 2009, researchers followed more than 11,000 Canadians over a 12-year period. They then calculated overall risk of death in each category (e.g. 'underweight', 'healthy', 'overweight' and 'obese').[2]

The results of this study showed that, compared to individuals in the 'healthy' category (BMI 18.5–24.9), overall risk of death for the other categories was as follows:

- underweight (BMI <18.5): 73 per cent increased risk of death

- overweight (BMI 25.0–29.9): 17 per cent *reduced* risk of death

- **obese (BMI 30.0–34.9): no statistically significant difference in risk of death.**

Here we find that the lowest risk of death overall was found in individuals classified as 'overweight'. Another surprise result from this study was that being 'obese' did not appear to put individuals at a significantly increased risk of death. In fact, a significant increase in risk of death was seen only once BMIs rose above a really quite hefty 35.

Another way to assess the relationship between BMI and health is to plot a graph of risk of death on one axis, against BMI on the other. This way it is possible to ascertain what BMI is associated with the lowest risk of death. Studies of this nature typically reveal J-shaped curves, meaning that both very low and very high BMI scores are associated with an increased risk of death. In one review, the results of 19 relevant studies were lumped together.[3] This review revealed that the lowest risk of death corresponded with a BMI of 25 (technically in the 'overweight' category).

Another similar study assessed the relationship between BMI and overall risk of death in almost 360,000 adults across 10 European countries.[4] In men, the low-point of the death curve in this study corresponded to a BMI of 25.3. Again, the evidence here suggests that, on a population basis, the ideal BMI falls in the 'overweight' category.

Now, these studies are based on populations and, the thing is, what we know about populations doesn't always apply to individuals. So, while a BMI of 25 might be ideal from a population perspective, that does not mean it's the best BMI for *you*. Remember, on an individual basis, the BMI tells us nothing about body composition. So, not only may the BMI not be a great guide to health, it is really quite useless for tracking the benefits you'll get from applying the information and advice contained in this book. I advise ignoring the BMI, as well as advice from well-meaning health professionals who tell you your BMI should fall in the 'healthy' category.

WHY WAIST?

At the start of this chapter we touched on the point that when we men gain weight, it tends to accumulate around our middles, and that it is this sort of fatty accumulation that appears to be most strongly linked with disease risk. Individuals who accumulate fat under the skin in the midriff also tend to be prone to deposition of fat *within* their abdomens, including in and around the organs here, including the liver. This type of fat – referred to as 'visceral fat' – is believed to be particularly hazardous to the body.

Over the last decade or so, doctors and scientists have given increasing attention to 'abdominal obesity', at least partly because of its links with chronic disease and ill-health. In fact, we have seen in relatively recent times the defining of a distinct medical condition – 'metabolic syndrome' – the cardinal feature of which is abdominal obesity.

While the exact definition of metabolic syndrome varies a bit according to whom you ask, there is general acceptance that its diagnosis depends on the presence of abdominal obesity accompanied by two or more of other common features associated with the condition.

- **Abdominal obesity**
  For the purposes of diagnosing metabolic syndrome, abdominal obesity is generally defined as a waist circumference of 94 cm (37 inches) or more for men.

The other features that are often used to establish the diagnosis of metabolic syndrome are:

- **Raised levels of triglycerides**
  Triglycerides are one type of fat that can circulate in the bloodstream. High levels of triglycerides are associated with an increased risk of heart disease. Triglyceride levels of more than 1.7 mmol/l (millimoles/litre) are generally regarded as elevated when metabolic syndrome is being considered.

- **Reduced levels of 'healthy' high-density lipoprotein (HDL) cholesterol**
  In most people's minds, cholesterol is viewed as a bad thing (more information about the relationship between cholesterol and health can be found in Chapter 4). However, it is widely accepted that one form of cholesterol – known as HDL-cholesterol – is associated with a *reduced* risk of cardiovascular conditions such as heart disease and stroke. Levels of less than or equal to 0.9 mmol/l are generally regarded as relevant when metabolic syndrome is being considered.

- **Raised blood pressure**
  High blood pressure is a risk factor for heart attack and stroke. A systolic pressure of more than 130 mmHg (pressure in torrs) and/or diastolic pressure of more than 85 mmHg is generally regarded as significant when metabolic syndrome is being considered.

- **Raised fasting blood glucose level or previously diagnosed type 2 diabetes**
  Type 2 diabetes is the most common form of diabetes, one of the features of which is an inability of insulin to function normally in the body – sometimes termed 'insulin resistance'. A fasting blood-sugar level of more than 5.6 mmol/l is generally regarded as significant when metabolic syndrome is being considered.

FATTY LIVER

Another potential feature of metabolic syndrome is a condition known as 'fatty liver'. This condition is characterised by, as its name suggests, deposits of fat within the liver. If left unchecked, fatty liver can lead to inflammation, fibrosis and even full-blown cirrhosis of the liver. For a long time it has been known that one dietary factor which can induce fatty liver and its later complications is alcohol. However, it is increasingly being recognized that fatty liver may have nothing to do with alcohol, and more to do with overconsumption of other foodstuffs. More about fatty liver and what dietary factors may drive it can be found in Chapter 3 (Carb Loading).

WHAT A WAIST

One way of assessing the extent of abdominal obesity is to measure the circumference of your waist. An alternative measurement is the waist-to-hip ratio (calculated by dividing the waist circumference by the circumference around the hips). Given the association between expanded waistlines and heightened disease risk factors, it's perhaps no surprise that big waists are associated with big problems for our health.

For example, large waist circumferences and high waist-to-hip ratios are associated with an increased risk of heart disease.[5] Abdominal obesity has quite a strong relationship with risk of death, too. For example, in the Europe-wide study mentioned above,[6] men with the highest waist circumferences had a more than two-fold increased risk of death compared to those with the lowest waist measurements.

BIG BELLIES MAY BE BAD FOR THE BRAIN, TOO

The evidence suggests that abdominal obesity is bad for the body, and other research suggests it might be bad for the brain in the long term, too. In one study, the relationship between abdominal obesity and risk of dementia was assessed over more than 30 years. Abdominal obesity was assessed by measuring the distance from the front of the belly through to the back (known as the *sagittal abdominal diameter*, or SAD).[7] The results of this study showed that individuals with the biggest SAD measurements were at an almost three-fold increased risk of dementia compared to those with the smallest.

If abdominal obesity does indeed turn out to increase the risk of dementia, how does it do it? Well, for a start, abdominal obesity is associated with an increased risk of cardiovascular disease, including stroke. Multiple, usually small, strokes in later life can cause parts of the brain to die off, and are clearly something that can compromise brain function (the medical term for this is 'multi-infarct dementia').

Another mechanism by which a big belly can affect the brain concerns blood-sugar balance in the body. Abdominal obesity, as we learned, is associated with metabolic syndrome, and in particular reduced ability to control blood-sugar levels. This is relevant because raised sugar levels can damage protein within the brain, effectively ageing this organ. This helps to explain why type 2 diabetes (characterised by raised blood sugar) and its precursor (known as 'impaired glucose tolerance') have been linked with impaired brain function in later life.[8]

Avoiding or reversing abdominal obesity and the biochemical imbalances that go with it could really help to preserve our mental faculties as we age.

TRACKING YOUR PROGRESS – WAIST CIRCUMFERENCE

We know that the BMI (or body weight) is a generally useless way to track changes in body composition and body fat levels. We also know that shedding belly fat is generally most important from an aesthetic perspective for most men, and is most relevant from a health perspective as well. With all this in mind, it makes sense for us to use waist size to keep tabs on our fat-loss progress over time. This can be done quite informally by, for instance, witnessing your ability to pull your belt in a couple of notches or finding yourself able to get into suit trousers you haven't been able to wear for some time.

However, if you want to be more precise about it, then tracking your waist circumference over time makes sense.

BELT UP – ONE MAN'S STORY

I'd never had much of a weight problem in my youth, but during my thirties the pounds just crept on. My problem areas were my belly and neck. I had a paunch and a double chin to match. For most of my adult life I had worn 30-inch-waist trousers. Eventually, I only felt truly comfortable in a 34. I decided to take action by getting my diet in order. We didn't have a set of scales in the house, so weighing myself was not an option. I did, however, set a goal of being able to get into 30-inch-waist trousers again.

Quite soon after changing my diet, maybe even within a couple of weeks, I found everyday trousers were feeling looser. A couple of months down the line and I was getting into stuff I hadn't worn in a while. Around this time I went away on business and took a belt I hadn't used for some time. When I put the belt on in the morning I realized that even on the tightest setting, it was now too big for my waist. I had to borrow a penknife from a waiter at breakfast to make a new hole in it. I ruined the belt, but I got a lot of satisfaction out of needing to make that new hole!

There is some debate about the best way to measure waist size, including precisely where the tape measure should go. What is really important, though, is not *where* you take this measurement, but that you take it in the *same place* each time. I advise measuring waist circumference at the level of the belly button, which serves as a useful landmark. You need to make sure the tape is horizontal with the ground all the way round (it helps to check this in a mirror or have someone help you with it).

Recommendations are usually to take the measurement on the out-breath. However, slack abdominal muscles lead to a bigger reading than tauter muscle tone here. This becomes relevant if your abs are currently slack, and you remedy this situation with some sit-ups (see Chapter 10). One way to counter this is to breathe out and also tense your abdominal muscles before you take the waist measurement.

Waist size is an important measure, but not one that you can expect to change on a day-to-day basis. For this reason, I recommend checking it no more frequently than once a week for the first few weeks, and less frequently thereafter.

TRACKING YOUR PROGRESS – BODY FAT

Some individuals like to monitor their progress by assessing body fat levels, too. The most practical way to do this is to measure the amount of fat under the skin (known as subcutaneous fat) at one or more points around the body using specially designed callipers. Commonly used sites include the waist, the back of the upper arm (over the triceps muscle), the front of the arm (over the biceps muscle), the chest (over the pectoral muscle), and front of the thigh. Skin folds are generally measured vertically or on the diagonal rather than horizontally.

Several measurements can be taken, and then a formula can be applied to convert these measurements into the total body fat percentage of the body. However, there are many different formulae, and even with the same skin-fold measurements, they can give quite different results. Basically, there is no one, single, correct way of assessing body fat percentage using skinfold callipers.

An alternative approach is to dispense with the idea of calculating body fat percentage, and just keep track of the calliper measurement scores either individually or totalled up. These simple measurements will give you a good indication of your fat-loss progress without the need for fancy formulae.

A lot of money can be spent on callipers, but there's really no need. The plastic callipers I have (Accu-Measure) cost a few pounds and do a good job. They come with the recommendation to measure just one site (2–3 cm above the front and top of the right pelvic bone). The callipers are accompanied by a chart which allows this one measurement to be converted into an overall body fat percentage.

Like waist circumference, body-fat calliper measure-ments do not change quickly over time, and I therefore recommend weekly measurements at most to begin with, and no more than monthly measurements in the longer term.

IF YOU MUST …

Despite the fact that measuring weight doesn't yield much useful information and is not much cop at tracking progress, some of us will find it hard to resist its allure. Scales are easy to use, and a good set can detect small changes that are harder to capture using waist and skinfold thickness measurements. Do bear in mind, though, that any loss in weight can be due not just to fat loss, but loss of other things including water and glycogen (a storage fuel found in the liver and muscles). This is particularly true in the early stages of any weight-loss programme.

Another thing to consider is that the body can be prone to quite significant fluctuations in weight which may not have much to do with what you've eaten, and this can be misleading. For example, on a hot, dry day we can quite easily drop a kilogram or so because of dehydration. Conversely, during a hot, low-pressure spell the body tends to retain more water, causing our weight to spring up. Because of the potential for day-to-day fluctuations, I suggest weigh-ins should be no more frequent than weekly.

If you are committed to weighing yourself, then the accuracy of this endeavour will be improved by using a decent set of scales. Electronic scales, many of which are relatively inexpensive, will generally do a good job. Put them on a hard, level surface for maximum accuracy.

BACK TO BASICS

- **The BMI is a pretty useless guide to health, principally because it tells us nothing about body *composition*.**

- **The BMI is not useful for tracking changes in body composition or fat loss.**

- **Excess fat around the middle (abdominal fat) appears to be toxic to body and brain.**

- Tracking your waist measurement is a good way to monitor your fat-loss progress.

- The use of body-fat callipers can be useful from this perspective, too.

Chapter 2

THE CALORIE TRAP

WHY COUNTING CALORIES
IS A WASTE OF TIME

For more than half a century, conventional weight-loss advice has been based on the calorie principle. Essentially, this states that if we consume fewer calories than the body burns (during activity and as a natural consequence of metabolism), weight loss will result. It is this principle that has led to the oft-quoted dictum that people who want to lose weight just need to 'eat less or exercise more'.

There is some truth in the calorie principle. After all, if you starve people, in the long term they most certainly will lose weight. However, despite decades of calorie-focused advice and an ever-expanding range of calorie-reduced foods at our disposal, rates of obesity are burgeoning. In the real world, the dominance of the calorie principle in our thinking has been a dismal failure.

When individuals fail to lose weight applying the calorie principle, there is a tendency to assume that they must be sneaking food in somewhere, or not being as active as they claim. But actually, the evidence shows that calorie restriction through dieting is simply not effective for *long-term* weight loss. Neither, by the way, is exercise (as we will explore in Chapter 10). On the face of it, there certainly seems to be a case for taking failed slimmers out of the dock, and putting the calorie principle in their place.

This chapter explores why calorie counting is so often a disaster for long-term weight loss. But don't worry – in subsequent chapters you'll learn the strategies that deliver lasting results on the fat-loss front.

IS A CALORIE A CALORIE?

A calorie is a unit of energy, which in the diet can come in different forms (i.e. carbohydrate, protein, fat and alcohol). When weighing up calorie balance in the body, most health professionals do not distinguish between different *types* of calories. In other words, the general view is that 'a calorie is a calorie', and that the form it comes in is quite irrelevant for the purposes of considering its impact on body weight.

However, let's think about this for a moment. Imagine putting charcoal briquettes and petrol onto a lit barbeque. Both fuels will burn, but petrol will burn much more quickly than the charcoal. Not only that, but petrol leaves nothing behind, while some of the charcoal may not combust as completely. Could the same be true for food within the human body?

One way of putting this theory to the test is to assess the weight-loss effects of diets that contain the same number of calories, but are made up of varying amounts of fat, carbohydrate and protein. If it's only the total number of calories that count, then diets that contain the same number of calories should have the same effect on weight, right? Actually, there is evidence that this is not necessarily the case.

One early study to examine this concept was published back in 1971 in the *American Journal of Clinical Nutrition*.[1]

A small group of young men (average age, 22) with an average body weight of almost 100 kg were asked to diet for 9 weeks. Each of the men was to eat 1,800 calories a day (about 2,000 calories less than they were accustomed to eating). The study subjects were split into three groups, with each group asked to eat a high-, medium- or low-carb diet (104, 60 and 30 grams of carbohydrate respectively each day).

Protein intakes were the same in each group, which meant that the men eating the most carbohydrate also ate the least fat, while those eating the least carbohydrate ate the most fat.

All groups lost weight, but the amount of weight lost was inversely proportional to the amount of carbohydrate in the diet: the less carb there was in the diet, the more weight was lost. Weight loss for high-, medium- and low-carb diets was an average of about 11, 12 and 15 kg respectively.

The researchers assessed *fat loss* in each group as well, which turned out to be about 8.4, 10.2 and 14.8 kg respectively. In short, the men eating the most fat were the ones who also *shed* the most fat from their bodies.

It is possible, of course, that the individuals who lost the most weight and fat did so because they were more active. Actually, though, activity was the same across the groups. The logical conclusion is that the differences in weight and fat loss were due to differences in dietary *composition*.

This study is not the only research which has found that diets of different composition can have very different effects on weight. In another study, for instance, the effects of two diets differing in terms of carbohydrate content were assessed in a group of post-menopausal women over a six-month period.[2] Each of these diets contained exactly the same number of calories, but while one had 58 per cent of calories coming from carb, the other had 35 per cent. Women in both groups lost weight but, tellingly, the women eating more fat and less carb lost significantly *more* (7.7 kg versus 4.7 kg).

Another piece of research pitted a diet based almost entirely on carbohydrate with one in which only half the calories came from carbohydrate, with the other half coming from almonds (a low-carb, high-fat food).[3] Again, both these diets contained the same number of calories. Over 24 weeks, the almond-eating group actually lost 50 per cent more weight (an additional 7 kg) than their carb-consuming counterparts.

What these studies show is that different *types* of calories can impact differently on body weight and fatness. Plus, these studies show that, calorie for calorie, higher-fat, lower-carb diets tend to be more effective for the purposes of weight loss.

One potential problem with these studies, though, is that we can't be absolutely sure what and how much the participants ate. Even if you were to hole people up in a hospital ward and feed them specific foods of known quantity, individuals would have to be under 24-hour surveillance for researchers to know what they ate (and in particular if other foods were sneaked into their diet). Also, individuals tend not to like to have their diet controlled for too long in this way, and therefore such studies simply may not go on long enough for any weight-loss difference to materialise.

One way round these issues is to study animals. The diets of mice, for instance, can be utterly controlled and very accurately measured. Plus, researchers can conduct studies for as long as the mice remain alive. One relevant study was published in the *American Journal of Physiology*,

Endocrinology and Metabolism in 2007.[4] In this study, mice were fed one of four diets:

1. Regular mouse food (chow)

2. A high-fat, high-sugar diet containing the same number of calories as diet 1

3. Regular mouse food but with calories restricted by 1/3 compared to diet 1

4. A high-fat, low-carb (ketogenic) diet containing the same number of calories as diet 1.

The mice had their body weights monitored for nine weeks. The results of this experiment showed that mice eating the regular chow and the high-fat, high-sugar diet (diets 1 and 2) gained weight. The mice eating the calorie-restricted diet (diet 3) lost weight. *However,* the mice eating the high-fat, low-carb (ketogenic) diet also lost weight. This despite the fact that they ate the same number of calories as the mice eating regular chow and high-fat, high-sugar diets who gained weight. The weight loss seen in these mice was about the same as that seen in the mice who had been given significantly less to eat.

The finding that high-fat, low-carb diets might have a weight-loss advantage is quite the reverse of what most of us have been led to believe. After all, fat, gram for gram, contains about twice as many calories as carbohydrate (and protein). So how could a low-fat, high-carb diet be less effective for weight loss than a higher-fat, lower-carb one? We'll be exploring potential explanations for such seemingly paradoxical results in subsequent chapters.

LOW CALORIE OFTEN MEANS LOW QUALITY

Another potential hazard associated with calorie-restricted eating is that it can cause us to eat a nutritionally inadequate diet. Just because something is low in calories, doesn't make it good to eat. Low-calorie diets can lead to a deficiency in key nutrients. For example, when fat is targeted as an offender, there is the risk that we can run short on what are known as 'essential fatty acids', including what are known as omega-3 fats, found in oily fish. These fats have a crucial role to play in health, and a deficiency in them can have negative consequences for both body and brain (this is covered in more depth in Chapter 4). A deficiency in omega-3 fats is just one example of the sort of dietary deficit we can run into if the quantity of what we eat takes priority over quality.

And low-calorie diets may not just cause us to miss out on key nutrients, they can also cause us to consume foodstuffs that can have adverse effects on health. For example, low-calorie dieters will often deploy artificial sweeteners in preference to sugar. While artificial sweeteners are promoted as healthy and safe, there is actually a lot of evidence which links their consumption with health issues including headaches and depression (more about this can be found in Chapter 8, Liquid Assets). And, as we'll see in Chapter 6 (Satisfaction Guaranteed), there is also evidence that artificial sweeteners can stimulate appetite and can, in time, actually *promote* weight gain.

CUTTING CALORIES CAN CUT THE METABOLISM, TOO

Those who preach from the calorie-principle bible often talk about calories consumed and calories burned, as if they do not influence each other. But they do. For example, in the chapter on exercise we'll explore how, when individuals step up their levels of exercise, their food intake tends to take a step up, too. Crucially, too, when calorie intake is reduced, this can put a dent in the metabolism.[5] If you don't put much fuel on a fire, it won't burn very well, and the body is no different.

Even when calorie intake is stepped up again, the metabolism may not recover in a timely fashion. In one study, calorie restriction was found to suppress metabolic rate.[6] However, even six months after the calorie restriction was lifted, metabolic rates were significantly lower than before the start of the study. It is this phenomenon that helps explain why after abandoning a 'diet', many individuals end up heavier than they were when they embarked on the diet in the first place. Talk about demoralising.

LESS IN MEANS LESS OUT

Another way that cutting back on calories may scupper long-term weight loss is through its impact on activity. Both of the last two studies discussed here found that when calories were restricted, individuals spontaneously moved less.[7] Of course individuals may be able to defy this in the short term by forcing themselves to stick to some exercise regime. Exercising more and eating less may well pay off in the short term. However, as some of us know all too well, this sort of regime can be mightily difficult to sustain in the long term. And a major reason for this has to do with *hunger*.

WHY HUNGER HAS NO PART TO PLAY IN SUCCESSFUL WEIGHT LOSS

If we swallow the calorie principle whole without thinking, we might imagine being hungry is a sure sign that we're in 'calorie deficit' and therefore *must* be losing weight. The problem with hunger, of course, is that it can sap the resolve and make changes quite unsustainable. While most of us can put up with intermittent hunger for a few days or even weeks, very few of us will be able to tough it out for any longer. What usually happens here is a return to the default diet, followed by an inevitable return of whatever weight that was lost, perhaps with some interest, too.

Also, it's important to bear in mind that different foods sate the appetite to differing degrees. Low-calorie foods often fail to satisfy us properly, which can make sticking with this approach nigh on impossible. On the other hand, even if a food is calorific, that won't necessarily matter if it has superior appetite-sating potential. Not only might this mean we don't eat too much of it, but it might lead us to eat less at a subsequent meal, too.

Long-term success will depend on eating the right foods, which at the same time do not leave us wanting more.

The following chapters will reveal precisely which these foods are.

THE PRIMAL PRINCIPLE – CALORIE COUNTING

A basic tenet of healthy eating, as we touched on in the Introduction, is that the best diet for the human species is a diet based on the foods that we have been eating for longest in terms of our time on this planet. Over the years there have been attempts to assess the diets eaten by indigenous 'hunter-gatherer' populations. Such diets are comprised ostensibly of natural, unprocessed foods including meat, fish, eggs, nuts, seeds, fruits and vegetables. The contribution each of these foods makes in the diet has been found to vary according to location. Further away from the equator, indigenous populations eat more animal and less plant foods compared to those living in warmer climes. However, whatever the precise nature of their diet, populations eating a 'primal' diet are untouched by obesity. And they don't count calories or concern themselves with portion sizes, either.

BACK TO BASICS

- The calorie principle has underpinned weight-loss advice for decades, and dictates that to lose weight we must eat less or exercise more.

- The calorie principle assumes that all forms of calories have the same impact on weight and fatness. Several studies show that this is not necessarily the case.

- Low-calorie diets can lack vital nutrients and can include foodstuffs that are toxic to health.

- Low-calorie diets can cause the metabolism to dwindle, which can make weight control harder in the long term.

- Low-calorie diets can leave us hungry, which can make them quite unsustainable in the long term.

- The secret to lasting fat-loss success is to eat the right foods that, at the same time, sate the appetite effectively.

Chapter 3

CARB LOADING

THE REAL REASON PEOPLE GET FAT

Carbohydrate in the diet comes in two principal forms – sugar and starch. We are generally encouraged to eat a diet rich in carbohydrate, including starchy staples such as bread, potatoes, rice, pasta and breakfast cereals. These are often promoted by health professionals because they supposedly provide valuable energy for the body, whilst being naturally low in fat. Wholegrain cereals such as wholemeal bread and brown rice get special recommendation because they have the added advantage of being rich in fibre and essential nutrients. No wonder, then, that starchy carbs form a cornerstone of our diets.

On the other hand, a vocal minority of doctors and scientists claim that excessive consumption of carbohydrates is at the root of the ballooning rates of obesity and ever-expanding waistlines. Dietary programmes such as the Atkins Diet, Protein Power and the South Beach Diet espouse 'low-carb' eating as a healthy way to lose weight and protect ourselves from chronic conditions such as heart disease and diabetes.

So, on the one hand some claim potatoes and grain-based foods such as bread, rice and pasta are the staff of life, while others see them as major causes of obesity and ill-health. So who is right? This chapter reveals the answer.

We're going to start by going over some physiology that is critical for understanding the impact carbohydrate has on weight and health.

FROM STARCH INTO SUGAR

Central to our assessment of the role carbohydrate-rich foods have on health is an understanding of the effect they have on the body's biochemistry and physiology. Sugar and starch may seem quite different, but actually they're pretty much the same thing. That's because starch is comprised of chains of sugar molecules. Once eaten, starch needs to be broken down in the gut into sugar before being absorbed through the gut wall into the bloodstream. This means that whether we eat sugar, starch, or a combination of both, blood-sugar levels will rise.

As levels of sugar in the bloodstream start to climb, the body brings into play mechanisms that are designed to keep them from rising too high. Key to this process is the hormone *insulin*, which is secreted by the pancreas. One of insulin's chief effects is to help transport sugar from the bloodstream into the body's cells. Without any insulin, sugar levels in the bloodstream would rise uncontrollably, with ultimately fatal consequences.

In this sense, insulin is essential to life, but, as with most things, you can get too much of a good thing. Excesses of insulin can have harmful effects in the body. One potential area of concern is the impact this hormone has on fat regulation in the body.

WHY WE GET FAT

In the last chapter (The Calorie Trap) we explored the idea that changes in weight are not solely determined by the balance of calories into and out of the body. We also learned how applying the calorie principle almost destines us to failure. The question is, is there a way of thinking about the processes that determine body weight that lead us to truly effective strategies for combating obesity?

Instead of viewing excess weight as a consequence of calorie excess, some scientists have suggested it might be useful to consider it as a disorder of 'fatty accumulation'. Could it be that there are certain circumstances in which the body tends to form and accumulate fat in a way that is, essentially, irrespective of calories?

This idea is explored in science writer Gary Taubes' best-selling book *The Diet Delusion* (entitled *Good Calories, Bad Calories* in the USA). In his book, Taubes considers the physiological and biochemical processes that drive us to have too much fat in our fat cells.

In the body, fat can circulate in the bloodstream in the form of what are known as 'free fatty acids', which can be burned to generate energy. Free fatty acids have the capacity to float in and out of fat cells, but only become 'fixed' in the fat cells once they are converted into a substance known as 'triglyceride'. Take a handful of the excess flesh around your midriff, and most of what you have between your fingers is triglyceride.

But what causes triglyceride to form in fat cells? Its raw materials come not just from free fatty acids, but another substance by the name of 'glycerol'. Glycerol is supplied from something known as glycerol-3-phosphate, which itself is derived from sugar (glucose).

So, the long and short of it is that sugar provides an essential element for the fixing of fat in the fat cells.

Most sugar in the body, under normal circumstances, comes from the consumption of carbohydrate in the form of sugar or starch. So, the more carbohydrate we eat, the more opportunity there is for fat to get stuck in our fat cells (and the fatter we get).

It is also perhaps worth bearing in mind that sugar's passage into the fat cells depends in the first place on insulin – a hormone secreted most plentifully in response to carbohydrate.

So, in summary, here is what can happen when we eat carbohydrate:

1. Glucose levels in the bloodstream rise.

2. Insulin is secreted.

3. Insulin stimulates the transport of glucose into the fat cells, where it can form glycerol-3-phosphate.

4. Glycerol-3-phosphate provides glycerol, which combines with free fatty acids to form triglyceride, essentially 'fixing' fat in the fat cells.

Clearly, insulin has a pivotal role in fatty accumulation. But its effects do not end there. Here are other known effects of insulin:

• activation of the enzyme *acetyl co-A carboxylase*, which stimulates the process known as lipogenesis (fat-production)

• activation of the enzyme *lipoprotein lipase*, which also stimulates lipogenesis

• inhibition of the enzyme *hormone sensitive lipase*, which inhibits the process of lipolysis (fat-breakdown).

In other words, insulin stimulates the accumulation of fat in the fat cells, and at the same time slows its breakdown.

Because carbohydrate is the primary driver of insulin secretion, then this macronutrient clearly has fattening potential. This concept is supported by studies in the scientific literature.

CARBOHYDRATE CONSUMPTION AND METABOLIC SYNDROME

In Chapter 1 (Toxic Waist) we explored a condition characterised by fatty accumulation around the midriff called 'metabolic syndrome'. What causes metabolic syndrome has been a subject of some debate, and the focus here has naturally been on dietary fat. Basically, the concept here is that eating a lot of fat is most likely to make us fat, and therefore increase our risk of the abdominal obesity that is the hallmark of metabolic syndrome. However, a common feature of metabolic syndrome is raised levels of insulin. Carbohydrate is the primary driver of insulin secretion. So, could it be that carbohydrate (not fat) causes metabolic syndrome?

In a study published in the *Journal of the American Geriatrics Society*, researchers went about assessing potential dietary risk factors for metabolic syndrome in a group of men aged 60–79 years.[1] This study showed that fat intake was not associated with metabolic syndrome risk, but carbohydrate *was*: the more carbohydrate individuals ate, the greater their risk of this condition.

Another potential feature of metabolic syndrome is what is termed 'fatty liver' (mentioned briefly in the first chapter). What causes fat to accumulate in the liver? In one study, the impact of diet on liver function and fat levels in the liver was tested in a group of healthy men and women.[2] The study participants were put on a regime which involved eating two fast-food meals each day for four weeks. Their results were compared with a group of individuals who were not subjected to the regime.

Over the course of the four-week study, there was biochemical evidence of significant liver damage, in the form of raised levels of the liver enzyme alanine aminotransferase (ALT). Not only that, but the fat level in the liver cells of these individuals increased by over 150 per cent (quite a feat in just four weeks). At the same time, body weight went up by an average of 6.5 kg.

It looks as though we have evidence here that gorging on fast food turns out to be bad for our weight and liver. But what was interesting about this study is that the authors looked at the relationship between different elements of the diet and changes in ALT levels. In other words, they wanted to see if they could find out what it was about fast food that seemed to have damaged the liver.

Here's what they found:

- Intake of *fat* was *not* associated with raised ALT levels.

- Intake of *protein* was *not* associated with raised ALT levels.

- Total calorie *intake* was *not* associated with raised ALT levels.

- Intake of *carbohydrate was*, however, associated with raised ALT levels.

Most imagine that the perils of consuming fast food relate to its ability to dish up unhealthy servings of fat. This study suggests that, as far as the liver is concerned, the truly toxic nature of fast food comes from carbohydrate.

Another reminder of the potentially toxic effects of carbohydrate on the liver concerns the making of *foie gras*. What is it that geese are force-fed to turn their livers into something that is almost entirely composed of fat? The answer is *grain*.

NOT ALL CARBS ARE CREATED EQUAL

We know that insulin is a key player in the development of obesity, and that carbohydrate is *the* chief driver of insulin production in the body. This puts carbohydrate firmly on the suspect list in terms of fattening potential. However, not all carbs stimulate the secretion of insulin to the same degree. How much insulin is produced after we eat, and our tendency to lay down fat, is linked with the speed and extent to which food releases sugar into the bloodstream. The blood-sugar-disrupting effects of foods can be measured and expressed as something known as the 'glycaemic index' or 'GI'.

One way of gauging the extent to which foods raise blood-sugar levels is to compare it to the body's response to consuming glucose (a very fast sugar-releasing food indeed). In the world of the GI, glucose is assigned a GI value of 100, and all other foods are compared to it. Basically, the higher a food's glycaemic index, the more disruptive its effects on blood-sugar and insulin levels are, and the more fat-making it will tend to be, too.

Just to give you a little flavour of how critical the GI of food can be, let's look at the results of an animal study which examined the impact of GI on fatty accumulation.[3] In this study, mice were fed either a low- or high-GI diet for a period of 40 weeks. At the end of the study, the mice that had been fed the high-GI diet had, overall, 40 per cent more body fat.

LOWERING INSULIN LEVELS IS THE KEY TO FAT LOSS

The bottom line: If you want to lose your belly fat easily and effectively, a key strategy will be lowering insulin levels in your body.

In this regard, restricting foods in the diet that cause surges in sugar and insulin makes perfect sense. What we need to know now, of course, is how disruptive specific carbohydrate foodstuffs are. Here's a list of some of the most commonly eaten carbohydrate foods and their GIs.

TABLE 1 Glycaemic indexes of various foods (adapted from Foster-Powell, K *et al.*, 'International table of glycemic index and glycemic load values: 2002', *Am J Clin Nutr* 2002; 76[1]: 5–56)

	Glycaemic index
Breads	
Baguette	95
bagel – white	72
wheat bread – white	70
bread – wholemeal	71
rye bread – wholemeal	58
rye bread – pumpernickel	46
bread – spelt, wholemeal	63
Crackers	
rye crispbread	64
cream cracker	65
water cracker	71
rice cakes	78
corn chips	63
potato crisps	54
popcorn	72
Pasta, rice and related foods	
brown rice	55
basmati rice	58
rice – Arborio (risotto rice)	69
rice – white	64
barley – pearl	25

pasta – corn	78
gnocchi	68
pasta – durum wheat	44
pasta – wholewheat	37
cous cous	65

Sweet foods

digestive biscuits	59
croissant	67
crumpet	69
doughnut	76
muffin – bran	60
scone	92
shortbread	64
ice cream	61
low-fat yoghurt	27
Mars bar	65
muesli bar	65
Snickers bar	55
honey	55
sucrose (table sugar)	68

Beverages

apple juice – unsweetened	40
cranberry juice	56
orange juice	50
Gatorade	78
tomato juice	38
Coca cola	53
Fanta	68
Lucozade	95

Breakfast cereals

All-Bran	42
Bran flakes	74
cornflakes	81

	Glycaemic index
muesli	40–66
porridge – home-made	58
porridge – instant	66
Special K	54–84
Shredded wheat	75
Raisin bran	61
Fruit	
apple	38
apple – dried	29
banana	52
mango	51
grapes	46
kiwi fruit	53
cherries	22
peach	42
pear	38
pineapple	59
plum	39
watermelon	72
figs – dried	61
apricots – dried	31
sultanas	60
raisins	64
prunes	29
strawberries	40
Legumes (beans, lentils, peas)	
baked beans	48
black-eyed beans	42
butter beans	31
chickpeas	28
hummus	6
kidney beans	28

lentils – green	30
lentils – red	26
peas – dried then boiled	22
peas – boiled	48
Vegetables	
peas – boiled	48
parsnips	97
potato – baked	85
potato – boiled	50
potato – new	57
chips (French fries)	75
potato – mashed	74
potato – instant mashed	85
yam	37
carrots – raw	16
carrots – cooked	58
pumpkin	75
beetroot	64

While there is continuing debate about how GIs should be classified, my preference is to call GIs of 70 or more 'high', GIs of 50–69 inclusive 'medium', and GIs of 49 or less 'low'.

What is important to know is that the many starchy carbohydrates are very disruptive indeed. Many of these staples, notably cornflakes, wholemeal bread and baked potatoes, have GIs even higher than table sugar (sucrose).

Look closely at the GI list and you will see that some fruits and vegetables, including beetroot, pineapple and watermelon, have high-ish GIs too. Does that mean that these foods are equivalent to foods with similar GIs such as corn chips and Mars bars? Actually, while the GI is an important measure, it's not the sole arbiter of a food's suitability for our consumption. How much we eat of that food is also critical. Foods with a relatively high GI will be most disruptive if we eat a lot of them. The eating of foods of high or medium GI matters less if we don't tend to consume too much of them at any one time.

Let's see how this may play out in real life. Imagine coming home ravenous and polishing off a bowlful or two of pasta in response. This is likely to cause considerable disruption in blood-sugar and insulin levels. On the other hand, it's highly unlikely that you would find yourself gorging on mounds of beetroot or pineapple for dinner, however hungry you were. When eaten, such foods tend to be eaten in very moderate amounts, and thus are unlikely to disrupt sugar and insulin levels much.

This concept has spawned the development of another measure of the effect of food in the body, known as the 'glycaemic load'. The glycaemic load of a food is calculated by multiplying its GI by the amount of carbohydrate contained in a standard portion of the food. This figure is then divided by 100. Basically, a food's glycaemic load (GL) is thought to give a more realistic guide to the impact of that food on blood-sugar and insulin balance.

While measuring GL values has some merit, the concept is based on standard portion sizes. However, people don't tend to eat 'standard portion sizes', so applying GL values listed in a table has little relevance to individuals in the real world. Looking at GL values does, though, help us gain some idea of how disruptive starchy carbs generally are in comparison to, say, fruits and vegetables.

Just as with the GI, what constitutes high or low is open to debate. But as a rough guide I recommend seeing a GL of 20 or more as high, and one of 10 or less as low. Anywhere in between can be classified as medium.

Considering GL values can cause a different picture to emerge than the one painted when judging foods by their GI alone. For example, many of the foods that have medium or high GIs turn out to have low GLs. Examples include kiwi fruit (GI 53, GL 6), pineapple (GI 59, GL 7), watermelon (GI 72, GL 4), cooked carrots (GI 58, GL 3) and beetroot (GI 64, GL 5).

On the other hand, the potato and many grain-based foods of relatively high GI have high GLs, too. Examples include bagels (GI 72, GL 25), white rice (GI 65, GL 23), rice cakes (GI 78, GL 17), cornflakes (GI 81, GL 21), baked potato (GI 85, GL 26) and pasta (GI 44, GL 21).

So, it's not just the fast sugar-releasing nature of the grain-based foods and the potato that poses problems for the body, but the fact that they tend to be eaten *in quantity*. Eating less of these foods will help to lower insulin levels, which promotes fat loss, pure and simple.

However, there is another major reason why eating less of these foods can be a boon for those wishing to shed fat. This concerns the impact that high-GI foods have on appetite.

THE EFFECT OF GI ON APPETITE

You may remember that in the last chapter (The Calorie Trap) the point was made that for long-term success, it's important to eat a diet that induces fat loss but not undue hunger. In a subsequent chapter (Let Them Eat Steak), we'll see that protein has particular value here. But what about carbohydrate?

Well, it turns out that, calorie for calorie, carbohydrate is less satisfying than protein. But it gets worse: the higher a food's GI, the less satisfying it is.[4] Overall, the results of studies in this area show that an increase in the GI by 50 per cent reduces the satisfaction it gives by about 50 per cent, even when calorie intake is the same. So, if you want to put a natural brake on your appetite, it really helps to eat lower-GI foods.

BLOOD-SUGAR IMBALANCE AND HUNGER

Why are high-GI carbs so useless for sating the appetite? One explanation has to do with the destabilizing effect these foods have on blood-sugar levels. The sky-high sugar levels these foods generally induce can cause insulin levels to surge. The risk here is that copious quantities of insulin will drive blood-sugar levels down to subnormal levels (a state known as hypoglycaemia). This is a major cause of hunger and food cravings, specifically for sugary, high-GI foods such as chocolate, biscuits, confectionery or soft drinks.

While episodes of low blood sugar can strike at any time of day, the most common danger time is mid- to late afternoon. A sandwich at lunch (perhaps coupled with a chocolate brownie or bag of crisps) is all that's required to cause blood-sugar levels to nose-dive in the afternoon.

HYPOGLYCAEMIA CAN PUT YOU TO SLEEP IN THE DAY, AND WAKE YOU UP AT NIGHT, TOO

False hunger and food cravings are not the only unfortunate side-effects of hypoglycaemia. Sugar provides ready fuel for the body, and if its supply stalls, fatigue is almost inevitable. The brain is particularly susceptible here because, although this organ makes up only about 2 per cent of our weight, it actually uses about a quarter of the sugar in the body at rest. If the brain is not adequately fuelled, it tends to malfunction. Common symptoms include poor concentration, loss of focus and sleepiness. Ever wondered why the mid- to late afternoon can find you devoid of energy and inspiration? It might have something to do with that sandwich, baguette or panini you ate at lunch.

Low blood sugar can affect mood, too. When blood-sugar levels drops, the body secretes hormones which stimulate the release of sugar from the liver. The chief hormone deployed here is adrenaline. That's fine on the football or rugby pitch, where it can be channelled appropriately, but may not be such as good thing if you're feeling stressed as a result of some situation at home or work. Tempers can fray.

Also, low blood sugar can occur in the night (after, say, a dinner comprised of pasta, ice cream and half a bottle of wine). Typically, blood-sugar levels will fall at around 3.30 or 4.00 a.m. As blood-sugar levels drop during the night, the body attempts to correct this by secreting adrenaline. Also, in response to low blood sugar the brain will ramp up its production of a chemical known as glutamate, which can cause feelings of agitation and excitability. This is obviously not ideal for restful sleep. Many individuals will be tripped into wakefulness, and often find it difficult to drop off again, too.

Stabilizing blood-sugar levels will help you stay awake during the day, stay asleep during the night, improve your mood and reduce any urge to eat foods you know are not the best for you.

LOW-GI OR LOW-CARB?

There is no doubt, I think, that eating a low-GI diet is healthier and more likely to induce fat loss and other health benefits than a higher-GI one. However, an individual eating a low-GI diet could still end up secreting a lot of insulin (and be at risk of the problems associated with this) if he eats enough carbohydrate. On the other hand, other macronutrients such as protein and fat cause less insulin secretion than carbs, and may therefore be better choices for those who have fat loss in their sights.

So, another way of being carb-conscious is to adopt a 'low-carb' diet. In practical terms, this means cutting down on, or possibly evening eliminating, starchy foods as well as those rich in sugar either naturally (e.g. honey, fruit juice, bananas, grapes) or unnaturally (e.g. chocolate, biscuits, muffins, confectionery, soft drinks). The precise definition of a low-carb diet varies, and some have suggested that diets containing 50–150 g of carbohydrate each day should be viewed as 'low-carb'.[5] Some dietary plans recommend even more carbohydrate restriction, particularly in their early stages. For example, the Atkins diet has an induction (initial) phase that permits a daily carb quota of no more than 20 g. Diets that restrict carb to this extent are generally viewed as 'very low-carbohydrate diets'.

I am a fan of low-GI diets. But if I were to choose between low-GI or low-carb for the purposes of fat loss, I'd opt for the latter. My experience in practice is that low-carb diets are really the most effective for shifting fat and improving markers of health. Plus, the science reveals low-carb regimes to be the most effective for weight loss (see below) as well as having the most favourable effect on measures such as fat, sugar and insulin levels in the bloodstream. For these reasons, the eating suggestions outlined in *Waist Disposal* are low-carb in nature.

WHAT DOES THE RESEARCH SHOW?

Low-carb diets should theoretically be effective for weight loss, and fat loss specifically. Studies assessing the effectiveness of low-carb diets have traditionally pitted them against the other major diet option – the low-fat diet. In many of these studies, those on a low-fat diet have been asked to intentionally restrict calories (typically 1,800 calories per day for men). On the other hand, those on the low-carb diet have generally not had their intake restricted. They are told to eat as much of permitted foods as they wish.

To date, seven studies have pitted low-carb against low-fat over various lengths of time. The shortest of these lasted three months.[6] The average weight loss on the low-carb diet was almost 10 kg. This compared very favourably with the weight loss on the low-fat diet, which averaged just over 4 kg.

The remaining six trials lasted at least six months.[7-12] All of these trials found that after six months, weight loss on the low-carb diet was significantly superior to that on the low-fat diet.

Four of the studies went on for a whole year.[13] Two of these studies[14] did not find a significant difference in weight loss between the two groups at the end of the study. In one study,[15] compliance was monitored, and it turned out that most participants did not cut their carb consumption to the level they were asked to. In another study,[16] there was no checking of compliance at all. In other words, it is just not known whether the study participants restricted carbohydrate to the extent they were instructed to. The two other year-long studies[17] did, however, find that the low-carb diet significantly outperformed the low-fat one in terms of weight loss.

To get an idea of the relative effectiveness of low-carb versus low-fat diets, we can tot up the average weight losses with each diet in all the studies, and divide this by the number of studies to get the average weight loss:

- **for the low-carb diets, average weight loss was 9 kg**

- **for the low-fat diets, it was 4.5 kg.**

Do you see a relationship here? Yes, that's right – overall, those on low-carb diets lost precisely twice as much weight as those slowly starving and depriving themselves on low-fat regimes.

And not only this, but low-carb regimes have been found to lead to more favourable outcomes with regard to, say, the lowering of triglyceride, sugar and insulin levels, and raising of 'healthy' HDL cholesterol.

IS THERE ANY OTHER EVIDENCE FOR THE EFFECTIVENESS OF LOW-CARB DIETS?

In a review of low-carb diets, weight loss where individuals ate 60 g or less carbohydrate was compared to that in individuals eating carbohydrate in greater quantities.[18] Lumping several studies together revealed that the average weight loss on the low-carb regimes was almost 17 kg, compared to less than 2 kg on regimes containing more carbohydrate.

Another relevant review looked at the impact of diets of different composition on several body measurements including weight loss, fat loss and body fat percentage.[19] Some 87 individual trials were included in the review. Lower-carbohydrate diets, compared to higher-carb ones, were found to bring about enhanced results in all the parameters assessed.

Specifically, in trials lasting 12 weeks or more, lower-carb diets led to:

- **an additional 6.5 kg in weight loss**

- **an additional 5.6 kg in fat loss**

- **an additional 3.5 per cent reduction in body fat.**

Taken as a whole, the research shows that low-carb diets are effective for weight and fat loss, and significantly outperform low-fat diets, too.

KETOSIS ON A LOW-CARB DIET

On a low-carbohydrate diet, about 70 per cent of the body's energy requirements will come from fat, including fat you're likely to be wanting to get rid of. A potential source of fuel is what is known as 'ketones', which can be made from both fat and protein. Perhaps the most famous 'ketotic' diet is the Atkins diet, which in its initial phase restricts carbohydrate to no more than 20 g per day.

Much has been made of the 'hazards' of ketosis. A good deal of this relates to the fact that it has a similar name to 'ketoacidosis', which can be induced in the body as a result of uncontrolled type 1 diabetes, and is viewed as a medical emergency. In reality, ketosis is a natural state which the body has adapted to switch on in times of food scarcity.

During ketosis, the body will generally be mobilising, and therefore losing, fat. That said, the body does not need to be in a state of ketosis to lose fat effectively. The dietary recommendations in *Waist Disposal* have not been designed with ketosis in mind. They have, however, been formulated for effective fat loss.

It is possible that, depending on your food preferences, you may enter a ketotic state from time to time while following the nutritional principles contained in this book. One risk here is that your body will 'cannibalise' protein (as well as fat) to make ketones. And one source of protein in the body is, of course, muscle.

There are three main strategies that can slow or stop muscle breakdown during ketosis (or indeed weight loss generally):

1. Eat a reasonable amount of fat, so that the body is less likely to need to look to protein for its source of ketones.
2. Eat a reasonable amount of protein, so that the body will look to this, not protein in the muscles, for its source of ketones.
3. Engage in regular resistance exercise to help preserve muscle mass.

Rest assured, the diet and exercise advice in *Waist Disposal* has all of these areas covered.

IS A LOW-CARB DIET BAD FOR THE HEART?

Despite the effectiveness of low-carb diets for weight and fat loss, they have managed to get themselves a pretty unhealthy reputation. A lot of this has to do with the fact that low-carb diets can be relatively rich in foods like meat and eggs. Conventional wisdom dictates that, on account of their saturated fat and cholesterol content, these foods have heart-stopping potential. We'll be looking at whether this belief is supported by the science in the next chapter (Fat Chance).

But another factor to consider here is whether high-carb diets are actually good for the heart. There's often an assumption that they are, but what does the research show? In reality, a body of research reveals that high-GI carb diets have the capacity to induce changes in the body that *promote* heart disease and stroke (cardiovascular disease).[20] Effects include:

- **increased 'oxidative stress' (also termed 'free radical damage', this is believed to be an important underlying factor in many chronic diseases including cardiovascular disease)**

- increased inflammation (which is emerging as a key underlying process in the gumming up of the arteries known as atherosclerosis)
- protein glycation (a process by which glucose binds to proteins in the body, damaging them)
- increased coagulation (essentially, making the blood 'stickier' and more likely to clot – something that can trigger heart attacks and strokes)
- raised blood levels of triglycerides (a known risk factor for cardiovascular disease).

Overall, the evidence links high-GI/GL diets with an increased risk of cardiovascular disease of between 20 and 100 per cent.

Other evidence linking carb consumption to cardiovascular disease came from a review published in 2009.[21] This very comprehensive review concluded that there is compelling evidence to suggest that high-GI/GL diets actually *cause* heart disease.

Remember that, generally speaking, low-carb diets have been found to induce favourable changes in triglyceride, sugar, insulin and HDL cholesterol levels, all of which would be taken as a sign of reduced risk of heart disease. One study found that after more than three years on a low-carb diet, subjects had 'relatively low values for conventional cardiovascular risk factors'.[22] This study provides good evidence regarding the safety of long-term carbohydrate restriction.

In short, the concept that low-carb diets are bad for the heart has no basis in science. If anything, such diets are likely to have benefits for cardiovascular health, while low-fat, high-carb diets look anything but 'heart-healthy'.

CARBOHYDRATES AND DIABETES

Another condition that is linked with carbohydrate intake is diabetes – a condition characterised by raised levels of blood glucose. It comes in two varieties: type 1 and type 2. Type 1 diabetes is caused by a lack of insulin produced by the pancreas. It tends to develop relatively early in life, and requires insulin for its effective treatment. Type 2 diabetes is usually caused by a 'numbing' of the body's response to insulin (referred to as 'insulin resistance'). It may also be caused by inadequate amounts of insulin levels due to what is known as 'pancreatic exhaustion'.

The more insulin we secrete over time, the greater the risk of both insulin resistance and pancreatic exhaustion. Seeing as carbohydrate is the dietary element that most stimulates insulin secretion, we might expect there to be a link between carbohydrate consumption and risk of type 2 diabetes. And indeed there is.

In one study, individuals with diets of the highest glycaemic load were found to be about 2½ times more likely to develop type 2 diabetes compared to those who consumed diets of the lowest glycaemic load.[23] Other evidence also links high-GI and/or -GL diets with increased diabetes risk.[24,25]

DEMENTIA

Excessive carbohydrate appears to have the potential for adverse effects on the brain, too. Studies in animals have shown that raised levels of sugar have the ability to damage a specific area of the brain that plays a role in memory (the dentate gyrus).[26] Raised blood-sugar levels will also increase the risk of something known as 'vascular dementia' (a situation caused, essentially, by narrowing and perhaps complete blockage in the vessels supplying blood to the brain). Risk of this goes up if metabolic syndrome or type 2 diabetes is present. As we discovered in the first chapter, abdominal obesity is associated with an increased risk of dementia.[27] If you're keen to keep your mind sharp as you age, then a low-carb diet may well help.

THE PRIMAL PRINCIPLE – CARBOHYDRATE

Evolutionists tell us that we've been on this planet some 2½ million years, and for the vast majority of this time we subsisted on a diet made up of meat, fish, eggs, nuts, seeds, fruits and vegetables. Up until about 10,000 years ago, we ate no grain at all. Things are very different now, of course. Grain-based foods such as bread, rice, pasta and breakfast cereals now account for about a third of the total calories we consume as a population.[28] And carbohydrate (of all forms) makes up 46 per cent of the calories we eat in total. In primitive hunter-gatherer diets, this figure averages out at about 30 per cent.[29] In other words, we are likely eating more carbohydrate than our bodies are adapted to eat. The forms of carbohydrate that we eat in the modern-day diet tend to be disruptive for blood-sugar and insulin levels, and are relatively low in nutritional value, too (see below). It is perhaps no wonder, then, that our carb-rich contemporary diet has the capacity to induce modern-day maladies such as obesity, heart disease and type 2 diabetes.

JUST HOW NUTRITIOUS ARE GRAINS, ANYWAY?

One common concern about the restriction of starchy carbohydrates such as bread and breakfast cereals in the diet is that, in doing so, we will be missing out on much-needed nutrients. However, while it's often taken for granted that grains, particularly wholegrains like wholemeal bread and brown rice, are packed full of nutrients, does this notion actually stand up to scrutiny?

One way to assess the nutritional value of a food is simply to measure the levels of key vitamins and minerals in it. While it makes sense for us to eat foods that offer a lot in terms of nutrients, some scientists believe that it helps to factor in the calorie content of these foods, too. The best foods would be judged to be those that have a combination of high nutrient levels and low calorie content. This has led researchers to develop a concept known as the 'nutrient density score'.

In a study published in the *American Journal of Clinical Nutrition*, the nutrient density of commonly eaten foods was assessed.[30] The nutrient density was based on the levels of 14 key nutrients (vitamins A, C, B_1, B_2, B_{12}, D, E, folate, calcium, iron, zinc, potassium, monounsaturated fat and fibre).

Figure 1 summarises the results for fruits and vegetables. The healthiest foods will generally be those that are positioned low and to the right on the graphs. Looking at this figure, we can see that fresh fruits and vegetables, with the exception of the potato, rate generally very well indeed.

Now compare these results to those obtained for grains, as seen in Figure 2. As you can see, generally speaking, grain foods are higher in energy density and lower in their nutritional offering. This includes wholegrain foods such as wholemeal bread.

And if wholemeal bread does not rate well, let's not get our hopes up for refined grains such as regular pasta, white bread and white rice. Compared to fruits and vegetables, many grain-based foods are really not very nutritious at all.

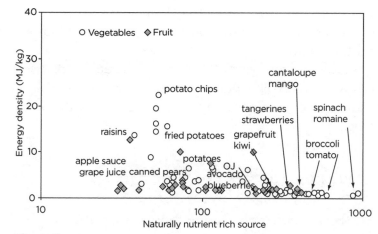

Figure 1

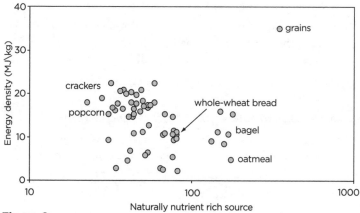

Figure 2

The bottom line is that while such fare is, strictly speaking, food, it is actually better described as *fodder*.

It's also worth bearing in mind that some grains, notably whole wheat, contains substances called phytates which actually *block* the absorption of nutrients such as calcium, magnesium, iron and zinc. So, not only do many grains lack much in the way of nutrients, they can actually stop us getting maximum nutritional value from other foods we eat them with.

Individuals following official advice by eating a diet rich in starchy foods like potatoes and grains run the risk of ending up overweight and malnourished, all at the same time.

WHERE'S MY ENERGY GOING TO COME FROM?

Another concern is that a low-carb diet will mean the body will run short on the sugar it needs to fuel itself. Sugar, in the form of glucose, is indeed a fuel for the body, and for some parts of the body (for example the red blood cells, and the lens and cells in the retina in the back of the eye) it is the *only* fuel. So, if carbs are cut, won't the body suffer? First of all, low-carb does not mean *no* carb. Even if the diet was completely devoid of starchy carbohydrate, some carbohydrate would still be available to the body from, say, fruits and vegetables.

But let's imagine for a moment that someone decided to eliminate every last molecule of carbohydrate from his diet, and eat nothing but protein and fat. What would happen then? The fact is the body has the capacity to convert both protein and fat into glucose. It has been estimated that about 200 g of glucose can be generated this way each day.

It is a plain and simple fact that the body's absolute requirement of carbohydrate is none at all.

This is, by the way, in stark contrast to fat and protein, as these supply elements that are essential to health (known as essential fatty acids and essential amino acids) which can *only be supplied via the diet.*

BACK TO BASICS

- Obesity can be viewed as a disorder of excessive accumulation of fat in the body.

- Insulin is the chief driver of fatty accumulation in the body, in that it promotes the deposit of fat in fat cells, while slowing fat breakdown.

- Foods that release substantial amounts of sugar into the bloodstream generally cause the body to secrete large quantities of the hormone insulin.

- In the short term, surges of insulin can cause blood-sugar levels to drop, which may provoke symptoms such as fatigue in the mid- to late afternoon, waking up in the night and cravings for sweet foods.

- In the long term, excess insulin can promote weight gain and increase the risk of conditions such as heart disease and type 2 diabetes.

- The extent to which a food destabilises blood-sugar levels can be measured, and is expressed as its 'glycaemic index' (GI).

- The overall effect of a food on blood-sugar and insulin levels will depend not just on its GI, but on how much of that food is eaten. This overall effect can be expressed as a food's 'glycaemic load' (GL).

- Many grain-based foods have high GIs and GLs.

- Lowering insulin levels is a key strategy for effective fat loss.

- Low-carbohydrate diets are effective for weight loss, and consistently outperform low-fat diets in this regard.

- Low-carb diets generally lead to favourable changes in fat, sugar and insulin levels in the bloodstream.

- With extreme carbohydrate restriction, the body can derive energy from ketones which can be formed from either fat or protein.

- Ketosis is not inherently damaging to the body, but can cause muscle loss. To mitigate against this, it is important to keep up a good intake of protein and fat, and to engage in resistance exercise.

- It is not necessary to be ketotic to lose fat effectively.

- Grains tend to have low nutritional value, even in their wholegrain form.

- The absolute dietary requirement for carbohydrate is actually none at all.

Chapter 4

FAT CHANCE

WHY EATING FAT ISN'T FATTENING

Conventional nutritional wisdom dictates that one of the keys, perhaps *the* key, to successful weight loss is to keep the diet low in fat. There is a widespread belief that eating fat is inherently fattening. This has something to do with its name (it is called *fat*, after all). But a lot of it relates to the fact that fat, gram for gram, contains twice as many calories as either carbohydrate or protein. The idea here is that if we eat a lot of fat, we run the risk of consuming calories that are surplus to requirements, and these will end up being dumped as fat in our tissues. On the face of it, those who promote low-fat diets for weight loss do seem to have a point.

On the other hand, we have the experience of countless individuals who, on a low-carb 'Atkins'-like diet, have had their fill of bacon and eggs, steak and butter, only to see their own internal fat melt away. Plus, we know that studies of such diets show them to be genuinely effective for weight loss. These observations should, if nothing else, cause us to question the widely-held belief that the fat we put in our mouths is somehow destined to end up in the fat stores in and around our body.

In this chapter we're going to look at the evidence regarding the role that fat plays in obesity. We'll also be looking at the different types of fat in the diet and the impact they have on health. First of all, though, we're going to see what evidence there is for the notion that fat is fattening.

IS FAT FATTENING?

While fat's calorific nature has been used to paint it as the most fattening element of the diet, we learned in Chapter 2 (The Calorie Trap) that the calorie principle is a gross oversimplification of what determines body weight and fatness. Thinking theoretically for a moment, there are several reasons why dietary fat may have been unfairly incriminated as a cause of body fatness. Here are the main ones:

1. **Not all calories have the same propensity to cause weight gain**

   In the second chapter we discovered that not all types of calories are necessarily metabolised in the same way, nor have the same propensity to cause weight gain. Actually, we learned that there is evidence that, for a given number of calories, higher-fat (and lower-carb) diets are generally the most effective for weight loss.

2. **Fat might help to sate the appetite, causing people to eat less overall**

   Fat stimulates the secretion of the hormone cholecystokinin, which slows the rate at which the stomach empties itself, and can prolong feelings of fullness. Studies have found that, for a given number of calories, fat can be more effective at sating the appetite than carbohydrate.[1, 2]

3. **Not all fat that is eaten is necessarily absorbed from the gut anyway**

   Studies show that when fatty food is eaten, not all of it gets absorbed into the body. Some ends up going straight down the toilet.

4. **Fat that is eaten doesn't necessarily end up getting stuck in the fat cells**

   In the last chapter we learned that, for fat to get fixed in the fat cells, glucose is required. Glucose principally comes from carbohydrate in the diet, and requires insulin to get into the fat cells, where it plays a key role in the manufacturing of fat. Remember, carbohydrate is the primary driver of insulin secretion in the body. So, in the absence of carbohydrate, it's theoretically very difficult for fat to get stuck in our fat cells.

So, in theory at least, there are a few good reasons why fat may not be all that fattening. One way to put this theory to the test scientifically is to assess the impact of eating fatty food on body weight. Let's use nuts as an example. About 80 per cent of the calories in nuts come from fat. They're about as fatty a food as we're going to find. But are they *fattening*?

The impact that nut-eating has on weight was the subject of an extensive review published in 2003.[3] This review showed that, generally speaking:

1. In populations, those who eat nuts generally weigh less than those who don't.

2. When people are fed nuts, they don't gain weight.

3. When individuals increase their nut consumption, many actually *lose* weight.

You may remember that in Chapter 2 (The Calorie Trap) we looked at a study which found that a diet rich in almonds led to significantly more weight loss than one without, even though calorie intakes were the same.[4]

An analysis of the relationship between nut-eating and body weight demonstrates that fatty foods are not necessarily fattening at all.

If eating fatty foods is not necessarily fattening, could it be that eating low-fat foods is not particularly slimming, either?

HOW EFFECTIVE ARE LOW-FAT DIETS FOR WEIGHT LOSS?

The acid test of the 'fat is fattening' theory is to put people on low-fat diets and see if they lose weight successfully in the long term. The best of such studies pit the low-fat diet against another diet that is calorie-controlled, but not explicitly low in fat (a 'control' diet). The results of several relevant studies were reviewed by an international group of researchers known as the Cochrane Collaboration in 2002.[5] The researchers were particularly interested in the ability of participants to sustain weight loss over a relatively long period of time.

The average amount of weight lost in low-fat and control diets were assessed at 6, 12 and 18 months. The following table summarises the findings of this review.

	AVERAGE WEIGHT CHANGE ON LOW-FAT DIET (KG)	AVERAGE WEIGHT CHANGE ON CONTROL DIET (KG)
6 MONTHS	- 5.08	-6.50
12 MONTHS	- 2.30	-3.40
18 MONTHS	+ 0.1	-2.30

You will see from this table that any initial weight loss enjoyed on a low-fat diet declines over time. This was also true of the control diets, but not nearly to the same extent. Plus, the control diets out-performed the low-fat diets at every stage. And perhaps most important of all, at 18 months, those instructed to eat low-fat diets had, on average, actually *gained* weight, while those eating control diets had lost some.

This study was withdrawn in 2008, on the basis that it was out of date, and that the authors had no intention of updating it. Back in 2002 the evidence clearly showed that low-fat diets are not effective for the purposes of weight loss, and the reality is that nothing has changed now.

So, weight loss on low-fat diets is nothing to shout about. What about *fat loss*? This question was considered by a major review conducted at the Harvard School of Public Health in the USA.[6] After reviewing literally dozens of studies which examined the relationship between fat-eating and body weight, as well as the effectiveness of low-fat diets, the authors concluded that 'Diets high in fat do not appear to be the primary cause of the high prevalence of excess body fat in our society, and reductions in fat will not be a solution.'

So, now you know – eating fat is not inherently fattening, and eating less of it is unlikely to help you in your quest to shed your spare tyre, either.

FAT FACTS

Fat in the diet comes in several different types including 'saturated', 'monounsaturated', 'polyunsaturated' and 'partially-hydrogenated' forms. Fats are composed of what are known as 'fatty acids' which, in essence, are made up of chains of carbon atoms with hydrogen atoms attached to them. The main classes of fat have subtle but important differences that distinguish them and their effects on health.

Saturated fats

The terms 'saturated', 'polyunsaturated' and 'monounsaturated' refer to the amount of hydrogen a particular fat contains. 'Saturated' fats, as their name suggests, contain as much hydrogen as they possibly can. This type of fat is found in animal products such as meat, eggs, butter, cheese, milk and cream, as well as in some non-animal foods such as coconut, palm, and palm kernel oils.

Monounsaturated fats

When a fat does not contain a full complement of fat, it is described as being 'unsaturated'. Hydrogen atoms go 'missing' from fats in pairs. When a fat is missing just two atoms of hydrogen, it is called a 'monounsaturated' fat. Foods rich in monounsaturated fat include olive oil, avocado and nuts and seeds. The consumption of foods rich in monounsaturated fats is generally associated with a reduced risk of cardiovascular disease.

Polyunsaturated fats

Polyunsaturated fats have four, six or any other multiple of two atoms of hydrogen missing. Polyunsaturated fats come in two main forms: these are known as 'omega-3' and 'omega-6' fats.

The main omega-6 fatty acid in the modern-day diet is known as 'linoleic acid'. Rich sources of linoleic acid include plant oils such as hemp, pumpkin, sunflower, safflower, sesame, corn, walnut and soya oil. Omega-6 fat also comes in the form of what is known as 'arachidonic acid', which is found in foods such as meat, fish and seafood.

The major omega-3 fatty acids in the diet come in the form of alpha-linolenic acid (from plant sources such as flaxseed) and fats known as eicosapentaenoic acid (EPA) and docosahexaenoic acid (DHA), found mainly in oily varieties of fish.

Partially-hydrogenated fats
These fats start out life as polyunsaturated fats and, as their name suggests, are then chemically processed to add some hydrogen.

The production of partially-hydrogenated fats can result in the formation of related fats known as 'trans fatty acids' or 'trans fats'. The word 'trans' refers to the chemical shape of these molecules. In general terms, these fats are a different shape to fats found naturally in nature, which usually have a different – 'cis' – shape. Partially-hydrogenated and trans fats can be found in processed foods such as chips, fast food (such as burgers and chicken nuggets), margarine, biscuits, cakes, pastries and crackers.

SATURATED FAT AND HEART DISEASE

Some argue that even if fat is not fattening, there is good reason to avoid certain fats because of their ability to induce heart disease. What people are usually referring to here is so-called 'saturated' fat found most plentifully in meat, eggs and dairy products (see 'Fat Facts', above). The idea that saturated fat causes heart disease was first floated back in the 1970s, when a researcher by the name of Ancel Keys found a strong association between the amount of saturated fat consumed and the risk of heart disease in seven countries.[7]

Studies like these seem, on the face of it, to be pretty convincing evidence that eating fat, particularly saturated fat, is a risk factor for heart disease. However, it's important to bear in mind that studies of this kind are what are known as 'epidemiological' in nature. This type of research essentially analyses the relationship between factors such as diet or exercise and health. The problem is, even if an association between two things is found, this does not prove that one is *causing* the other. For example, studies have found that *owning* a car is associated with an increased risk of heart disease. It's unlikely, though, that just owning a car actually *causes* heart disease. More likely it's other factors associated with car ownership, such as a tendency to be less physically active, that are the true causative factors. So, even if a study shows an *association* between saturated fat intake and heart disease, it cannot be used to conclude that saturated fat actually *causes* heart disease.

Also, while Keys' work is commonly cited as evidence that saturated fat causes heart disease, it focused on only a handful of countries. When a wider look is taken to include many more countries, the association found by Keys just disappears. Plus, Keys' study was just one study from more than 30 years ago. What does other evidence show?

There have, to date, been more than two dozen studies which have analysed the relationship between saturated fat and the risk of heart disease.[8-33] All but four of these studies[34] found no apparent association. And in one study, higher intakes of saturated fat in the diet were found to be associated with *reduced* narrowing of the arteries supplying blood to the heart (the coronary arteries) over time.[35]

Taken as a whole, the scientific evidence simply does not support the notion that saturated fat is bad for the heart. And remember, even the scant evidence that exists which supports a link is 'epidemiological' in nature, which may show an association, but does not prove that saturated fat causes heart disease.

In order to ascertain whether saturated fat might actually cause heart disease, what we need is what are known as 'intervention' studies. This essentially means putting people on a diet low in saturated fat in the long term to see what effect this has on their risk of heart disease.

To date, there have been more than 20 such studies,[36-57] of which just six[58] found benefit in terms of lower risk of heart disease. The evidence looks even less convincing when you consider that the studies that *did* find benefit are often what are known as 'multiple intervention' studies – which, in this case, means that in addition to reducing saturated fat, the participants in these studies were subjected to at least one other modification. For example, in one study individuals were given nutritional supplements. In other studies individuals were asked to emphasize heart-healthy omega-3 fats as well as fruit and vegetables in their diet. The obvious question that multiple intervention studies raises is whether lowered saturated fat in the diet, or the other interventions, or a combination of these things, was what proved effective. Because of these limitations, multiple intervention studies cannot be used to judge the effects of reducing saturated fat in the diet.

One way researchers can get a good idea of the overall effect of some treatment or approach is to perform what is known as a 'meta-analysis'. Here, results from a number of similar studies are grouped together. The largest meta-analysis to examine the effect of modifying fat in the diet was conducted by UK-based researchers and was published in the *British Medical Journal*.[59] This particular review amassed the data of 27 individual studies. Neither deaths due to cardiovascular disease (such as heart attack and stroke) nor overall risk of death was found to be reduced by making changes to one's intake of dietary fat. Cardiovascular 'events' (e.g. heart attack and stroke) were not reduced either. The results of this review support the notion that eating less saturated fat has little, if any, benefits for our heart and general health.

The most recent review of the role of saturated fat in heart disease was conducted by a group of researchers from McMaster University in Canada.[60] They undertook what is known as a 'systematic' review of the evidence, linking a wide variety of nutritional factors and heart disease. The authors of this review looked at evidence from both epidemiological and intervention studies. Here, in summary, is what they found:

1. **The epidemiological evidence does not support a link between saturated fat and heart disease.**

2. **There are no properly conducted intervention studies that support the notion that saturated fat causes heart disease, either.**

Eating less saturated fat is generally regarded as a key to good health. However, low-fat eating has not been shown to be effective for the purposes of weight loss in the long term, or for protecting us from disease. It appears there really is no point to eating a diet specifically low in animal fat.

It is, of course, possible to over-consume saturated fat. A diet, say, made of nothing but butter would not be a healthy one. Such a diet would lack the nutritional variety necessary for good health. By the same token, though, a diet based on broccoli would not be a healthy one either. The important thing here is that saturated fat is not inherently unhealthy, and therefore most certainly has a place in a healthy diet.

THE PRIMAL PRINCIPLE – SATURATED FAT

The evidence shows that there's nothing to be feared in saturated fat. Does its suitability as a food tie in with evolutionary theory? Well, saturated fat is a constituent in red meat. We've been on this planet about 2½ million years, and there is good evidence we have been eating meat for the whole of our evolution. How long have we been eating saturated fat for? The answer is *forever*. It really is something we should be quite well adapted to by now.

SATURATED FAT AND CHOLESTEROL

Those who believe that saturated fat causes heart disease will often cite the fact that this fat can raise blood-cholesterol levels. We are told that raised levels of cholesterol increases the risk of atherosclerosis – the artery-clogging process that increases our risk of so-called 'cardiovascular' conditions including heart disease.

There is indeed some evidence that high cholesterol levels are associated with an increased risk of heart disease and death, though a close look at the available evidence shows that this association only seems to be true for individuals up to the age of about 50 or so. After that time, plenty of evidence shows that 'raised' cholesterol levels in later life are not associated with adverse effects on health.[61-77] Indeed, there is even some evidence that higher cholesterol is actually associated with enhanced longevity and survival.[78-79] It should also be borne in mind that low levels of cholesterol are associated with an enhanced risk of death, principally as a result of an increased risk of cancer.[80]

As with saturated fat, if we really want to make a judgement of the true impact cholesterol has on health, we need intervention studies – studies in which cholesterol levels are lowered and the health effect of this assessed. In 2005 a review of 17 studies in which subjects made dietary changes explicitly to reduce blood-cholesterol levels was published in the *Archives of Internal Medicine*.[81] Overall, these studies brought about a 10 per cent lowering of cholesterol levels. Despite this, the amassed results showed no reduced risk of death in healthy individuals, nor in high-risk individuals who had already exhibited evidence of cardiovascular disease.

Evidence to date simply does not support the concept that taking dietary steps to reduce cholesterol has broad benefits for health.

IS MARGARINE REALLY BETTER THAN BUTTER?

For some decades now, margarine has been marketed as a 'healthy' alternative to butter. Initially margarine was sold to us on the basis that, compared to butter, it is lower in saturated fat. This selling proposition obviously rests on the assumption that saturated fat is bad for health. In this chapter, though, we have learned that there really is no good evidence that saturated fat is harmful to health.

The other claim made for some types of margarine, as we have just discussed, is that they help reduce cholesterol levels. Even if cholesterol reduction through dietary means had been proven to be beneficial (which it has not), would that mean something that *reduces* cholesterol is automatically healthy? It's the impact of a substance on *health* (not cholesterol levels) that is really important. Before we look at this, it's worth while thinking about where margarine actually comes from.

The major constituents of margarine are 'vegetable' oils, obtained from foods such as sunflower seeds, rapeseed or soybeans. These oils are usually extracted using the application of pressure and heat, and maybe the use of solvents, too. This processing can damage the fats and impart some unhealthy properties to them. The oil obtained by this process is then treated with sodium hydroxide to 'neutralise' certain fats in the oil that are unstable and may cause spoilage. After this, the oil is then bleached, filtered and steam-treated to produce what is essentially a colourless, flavourless liquid.

To convert this into margarine, this oil is subjected to chemical processes such as 'interesterification' or hydrogenation. Interesterification involves the use of high temperature and pressure, along with enzymes or acids, to 'harden' the oil. In hydrogenation, hydrogen is bubbled through the oil at high temperature. Both these processes have the potential to make fats that are unknown – something that should give us considerable cause for concern with regard to their effects on our health.

After this, the solidified fat that we now have is generally blended with other fats, which can be of vegetable or animal origin. And then the product needs to be both coloured and flavoured. Then what are known as 'emulsifying agents' are added to prevent the product from separating out. And finally, the end result is extruded into a plastic tub, for our delectation and delight.

Compare margarine's distinctly alien-to-nature nature to butter, which is made from the fat found in milk.

Half of butter's weight comes from saturated fat, while about 20 per cent of it comes from monounsaturated fat (believed to have positive heart-healthy properties). Apart from the addition of some salt, butter is a relatively natural, unprocessed food. We have not been eating it very long, but its constituents are found naturally in the diet.

So, what does the science show? One study in the scientific literature examined the association between butter and margarine consumption and the risk of heart disease in men.[82] This study found that butter consumption was not associated with heart disease risk. In other words, those men eating more butter were not at increased risk of suffering from heart disease. On the other hand, margarine consumption was associated with an increased risk of heart disease: in the long term, for each teaspoon of margarine consumed each day, risk of heart disease was found to be raised by 10 per cent. Other evidence links margarine consumption with a heightened risk of heart disease.[83]

It really should come as no surprise that a heavily processed, chemicalised non-food might turn out to have links with adverse effects on health.

THE HEALTH EFFECTS OF POLYUNSATURATED FATS

In contrast to saturated fat, polyunsaturated fats have been generally promoted as good for health, and for the heart in particular. These fats come in two main forms in the diet: omega-6 and omega-3 (see 'Fat Facts', pages **57–9**).

Omega-3 fats, found most abundantly in fish such as salmon, trout, mackerel, herrings and sardines, have been heartily promoted on account of their apparent health-giving effects. These fats have the capacity to thin the blood, reduce blood pressure and help maintain a normal heart rhythm – all things that would be expected to translate into reduced risk of heart attack, stroke and a condition known as sudden cardiac death. One review of 50-odd studies concluded that omega-3 fats, either from oily fish or fish oil supplements, have the capacity to reduce death rates due to heart disease, as well as overall risk of death.[84]

Omega-3 fats seem to have benefits for the brain, too. DHA is believed to play an important part in the structure of the brain. Higher levels of this fat in the body have been linked with a reduced risk of dementia.[85] EPA appears to contribute to the day-to-day running of the brain. Higher levels of this fat are believed to help ward against a variety of ills including depression, dyslexia and hyperactivity.

Both of these forms of fat can transform in the body into hormone-like substances known as eicosanoids (pronounced 'eye-coz-ah-noids'). Eicosanoids that come from the omega-6 fats tend to encourage physiological processes such as inflammation, blood-vessel constriction and clotting in the body.

Within the body, eicosanoids from omega-6 fats are balanced by the effect of those from omega-3 fats (e.g. the fats found in oily fish). The eicosanoids derived from omega-3 fats, generally speaking, tend to be anti-inflammatory in nature, and they have blood vessel-relaxing and blood-thinning effects, too. Because omega-6 and omega-3 fats have broadly opposing actions within the body, a 'balance' between these fats is vital for optimal health.

A glut of omega-6 fat in the modern-day diet may have important implications for our health. The higher the ratio of omega-6 to omega-3, for instance, the higher the risk of cardiovascular conditions such as heart disease and stroke.[86] Other evidence points to a raised omega-6:omega-3 ratio as a potentially important underlying factor in type 2 diabetes.[87] This fatty imbalance has also been implicated in inflammatory conditions and autoimmune disease – conditions where the body's immune system reacts against its own tissues, such as rheumatoid arthritis.[88]

A major source of omega-6 fats is refined vegetable oils, which make their way into our food supply in foods such as margarine, fast food and processed foods such as biscuits, cakes, pizza and pastries, and savoury snacks such as crisps, pretzels and corn chips. The evidence suggests that the dramatic increase we have seen in our intake of omega-6 fats is a potent force in the rise of many common health issues we now see in industrialised countries. Eating less of these foods will probably have benefits for health, as will eating more omega-3 fats to balance their effect.

THE PRIMAL PRINCIPLE – THE OMEGA-6:OMEGA-3 RATIO

Our ancient diet did indeed contain foods rich in omega-6 fat, such as meat, fish and nuts. However, only relatively recently did we start to consume much higher quantities of this type of fat in the form of cooking oils and fast and processed foods. Also, in our primal past we generally ate more in the way of omega-3 fats. It is estimated that the primal diet contained an omega-6:omega-3 ratio of about 1-3:1.[89,90] However, the fact that we are generally eating far more in the way of omega-6 fats and, almost certainly, less omega-3 too, has led to this ratio increasing to between 10:1 and 30:1 in a typical Western diet.[91] The imbalance in omega-6 and omega-3 consumption seen in the modern-day diet is believed by some scientists and nutritionists to be a factor in the development of conditions such as heart disease and arthritis.

A LOW OMEGA-6:OMEGA-3 RATIO CAN HELP BOOST FAT-BURNING

There is evidence that a lower omega-6:omega-3 ratio might help fat-burning in the body. In one study, individuals were asked to cut back on their omega-6 consumption, and at the same time eat three meals containing oily fish (rich in omega-3 fat) each week. In addition, they were asked to supplement with rapeseed oil at a dose of 20 ml a day, which provided them with a reasonable dose of the omega-3 fat alpha-linolenic acid.[92]

Before and during the study, the researchers measured a variety of disease-markers in the study subjects. Notably, dietary intervention led to a statistically significant increase in a substance known as adiponectin. This· hormone is secreted by fat cells, and has been shown to have generally beneficial effects on the body's physiology, including an anti-inflammatory effect and an ability to stimulate the breakdown of fat in the body. Interestingly, this study found that the prescribed diet led to a boost in the rate at which the subjects burned fat. In the fasted state, fat-burning was boosted by 28 per cent.

PARTIALLY-HYDROGENATED AND TRANS FATS

The increasing amount of omega-6 fats in the diet is not the only change we have experienced in our fatty intake in recent times. Another shift has been in our intake of so-called 'partially-hydrogenated' fats. These fats are unknown in nature, and have only made their way into our mouths since the processing of vegetable oils began in a big way just a few short decades ago. The hydrogenation of fats allows vegetable oils (such as sunflower and safflower oil) to be solidified, which is obviously critical in the manufacturing of solid fats such as margarine. The other 'benefit' of hydrogenation is that it makes fats less liable to turn rancid (go off), effectively extending their shelf life.

Again, evolutionary theory would suggest that foods containing partially-hydrogenated fats would *not* make particularly good choices from a health perspective. In the last decade or so, scientists have focused their attention on the health effects of a particular type of partially-hydrogenated fat known as 'trans fatty acid' or 'trans fats'. These fats are not only partially hydrogenated, but have also undergone an unnatural change in their molecular shape. As expected, the research suggests that industrially produced trans fats have the potential for wide-ranging unwanted effects on health.

TRANS FATS AND WEIGHT

There has not been much work which has examined the effect of the consumption of trans fats on body weight in humans. However, in one study, the effect of trans fat on monkey mass was assessed.[93] Here, one group of monkeys was fed a diet which contained 8 per cent of calories from trans fat. In another group of monkeys, these trans fat calories were replaced with naturally occurring monounsaturated fat.

All monkeys in the study were fed the same number of calories each day for a period of six years. At the end of the study, monkeys fed trans fat gained more than 7 per cent in body weight, compared to less than 2 per cent for the monkeys fed monounsaturated fat. Also, the trans-fat-fed monkeys tended to accumulate their weight in and around the abdomen – precisely the form of weight gain that we know is most strongly linked with conditions such as heart disease and diabetes.

Remember, these monkeys ate *the same number of calories*. This study provides further evidence for the notion that the *form* calories come in can have a profound influence on the effect they have on our weight and health.

TRANS FATS AND HEALTH

Trans fats have also been associated with adverse effects on health, including an increased risk of heart disease,[94-97] cancers of the breast and colon[98] and type 2 diabetes.[99-101] It's clear that industrially produced partially-hydrogenated and trans fats are well worth avoiding.

BACK TO BASICS

- While fat is often assumed to be fattening, there are a number of reasons why this is not necessarily so. Fatty foods may sate the appetite effectively and induce little in the way of insulin secretion (the chief driver of the accumulation of fat in the body).

- Low-fat diets have been shown to be ineffective for the purposes of weight loss in the long term.

- Saturated fat does not have a strong link with heart disease, and eating less of it does not have broad benefits for health either.

- Taking dietary steps to reduce cholesterol levels does not have broad benefits for health.

- There is no evidence that margarine is healthier than butter. Actually, evidence links margarine consumption with an *increased* risk of heart disease compared to butter.

- Omega-6 and omega-3 fats have antagonistic actions in the body, and having the correct 'balance' of these fats is important for optimum health.

- Generally speaking, reducing omega-6 intake and increasing omega-3 consumption is likely to bring benefits for health.

- Heavily processed fats known as partially-hydrogenated and 'trans' fat have a number of adverse effects on health and should be avoided.

Chapter 5

LET THEM EAT STEAK

WHY PROTEIN IS KEY FOR FAT-LOSS SUCCESS

Once upon a time, protein was seen as a supremely healthy part of the diet. It is, after all, known to be essential for growth, repair and regeneration in many body tissues, including muscle and skin. It also provides the raw materials for neurochemicals in the brain which are essential for optimal mood, focus and concentration, as well as being the basis for enzymes that catalyse thousands upon thousands of chemical reactions in the body intrinsic to health and life itself.

These days, though, protein tends to be referred to in quite negative terms. It's not uncommon, for instance, to hear that protein 'puts stress on the kidneys', or that it's bad for our bones. Some have even suggested that protein, specifically animal-derived protein, might be a potent force in the development of heart disease. It certainly seems as though protein has seen a quite spectacular fall from grace in recent times.

In this chapter we're going to examine the role that protein plays in health, and what place it has in our diet. We're going to start by examining the impact dietary protein has on what is likely to be your most pressing concern – the weight and composition of the body.

PROTEIN AND THE 'METABOLIC ADVANTAGE'

The chief function of the body's metabolism is to generate energy from food. Maintaining the metabolism is key to successful fat loss in the long term. Exercise is often said to boost the metabolism (more about this in Chapter 10), but another way to achieve this end with much less effort is simply to *eat*. Eating boosts the metabolism in a way that is similar to putting dry wood on an open fire. This phenomenon is referred to as the 'thermogenic' effect of food.

The thermogenic effect of food varies across different types of food. It turns out that protein has a significantly greater effect here than either carbohydrate or fat. When protein is eaten, it requires a fair amount of processing in the body that, if you like, burns calories for free. Some 20–35 per cent of the calories protein contains are metabolised this way.[1]

This increased thermogenic effect of protein compared to carbohydrate and fat has led some researchers to suggest that high-protein diets have a 'metabolic advantage'. In other words, for a given number of calories, higher-protein diets will lead to brisker weight loss because of their metabolism-boosting effects. Is there any evidence for this?

In one study, individuals were fed diets containing relatively high or low levels of a protein, derived from milk, known as casein.[2] Calorie intake was the same for each group. Individuals spent 36 hours living in a 'respiration chamber', which allowed analysis of energy expenditure and metabolic rate. The higher-protein diet, compared to the lower-protein one, led to higher total energy expenditure.

Other studies have measured the amount of energy a higher-protein diet burns over and above that of a lower-protein diet containing the same number of calories. The results of these experiments vary quite a lot, and range from about a 25-calorie difference over a 24-hour period, to a 60-calorie difference over 9 hours. These differences are small, but it is theoretically possible that small differences might lead to big benefits in the long term.

For the sake of argument, let's imagine that the additional calorie burn on a protein-rich diet is 40 calories per day. That equates to 14,600 calories over the course of a year. There are 9 calories in a gram of fat, which means the potential fat-loss advantage here is about 1,600 g or 1.6 kg (about 3.5 lb). We don't actually know if this benefit would materialise in reality, or if it would mount up over time, but there is at least some potential here.

Another potential benefit of protein is the fact that, well, it's *not* carbohydrate. This is relevant because carbohydrate is the chief driver of the hormone insulin, which, as we discovered in Chapter 3, has a big role to play in fatty deposition in the body.

However, whether the low-carb nature and metabolism-boosting effects of a high-protein diet offer a significant metabolic advantage is not particularly important, in my opinion. That's because protein offers a much more potent weapon in its arsenal in the fight against flab ...

PROTEIN – THE TASTE THAT FILLS

In Chapter 2 (The Calorie Trap) we explored how hunger has the capacity to scupper any attempts to shed fat in the long term. We have also touched on the notion that feeling properly satisfied by the food we eat is key to successful weight loss in the long term. Because different foods sate the appetite to different extents, it makes sense to emphasise those foods that are truly filling. It turns out that protein performs supremely well on this count.

Evidence to this effect comes from studies in which individuals have been fed a meal rich in protein, after which ratings of satisfaction were assessed. On another occasion, those individuals were fed a meal rich in carbohydrate and/ or fat containing the same number of calories as the high-protein meal. More than a couple of dozen such studies have been conducted now. The great majority of them have found that protein-rich meals are most satisfying.[3]

The mechanism behind the appetite-sating power of protein was investigated in a study published in the *Journal of Clinical Endocrinology and Metabolism*.[4] The study involved giving individuals beverages of different nutritional make-up. The beverages differed in terms of the relative amounts of protein, fat and carbohydrate they contained.

Before and after consuming the drinks, the subjects had their blood analysed for levels of a hormone called 'ghrelin' – higher levels of which are known to stimulate the appetite. Of all the food types tested, protein was found to be the best suppressor of ghrelin. It was also, not surprisingly, the most effective in terms of sating the appetite.

DOES THE EFFECT LAST?

Another way to test the effect of protein on satiety is to measure its impact on subsequent hunger and food intake. Here, researchers can give individuals a protein-rich meal and then measure how much they eat some hours later when given access to, say, a free buffet. On another occasion, the process can be repeated starting with a meal lower in protein.

A few of these studies have used methods that do not reflect eating behaviour in the real world. For example, in some studies individuals have been given liquid rather than solid food for the test meal. In others, noseclips have been used to mask the smell and flavour of the food (smell affects taste, and both these senses can influence satisfaction). Once such inappropriately designed studies are put to one side, the majority of studies show that eating a meal relatively rich in protein leads to reduced food intake at a subsequent meal compared to a meal of a lower protein content.

In summary, here's what we know about the effect of protein as it relates to weight control:

1. **Protein, compared to fat and carbohydrate, leads to a small but potentially significant boosting of the metabolism.**

2. **Protein sates the appetite more effectively than either carbohydrate or fat.**

3. **A higher-protein meal generally leads to less food being eaten later on.**

So, all this could lead one to believe that higher-protein diets are going to be generally effective for the purposes of weight loss. The question is: Does protein really deliver on its fat-loss promise?

THE EFFECTS OF PROTEIN-RICH DIETS ON WEIGHT LOSS

Several studies have assessed the impact of protein content in the diet on weight. In one such study,[5] individuals were first of all prescribed a calorie-controlled diet with protein making up 15 per cent of calories. After this, the diet was changed to one that contained twice as much protein.

The researchers found that, despite the fact that both diets contained the same total number of calories, the higher-protein diet led to significantly increased feelings of fullness and reduced hunger compared to the lower-protein diet.

The subjects in this study were then instructed to continue to eat this higher-protein diet for a further 12 weeks, but this time no restriction was placed on quantity. During this phase, individuals quite naturally ate less overall, and lost an average of 5 kg in weight.

A good judge of the effects of a high-protein diet on weight loss is to compare higher- and lower-protein diets side by side in a group of individuals. Most studies lasting a significant length of time have found that more weight is lost on higher-protein diets. For example, in one study lasting six months, a high-protein diet led to an average weight loss of 5.8 kg, compared to just 1.9 kg in a group eating a lower-protein diet.[6] In another six-month study, a higher-protein diet led to an 8.8-kg loss of weight compared to a 5.1-kg loss in individuals eating a lower-protein diet.[7]

This last study tested what is known as *ad libitum* diets, which means individuals could eat as much as they liked of the recommended foods. Those eating the high-protein diet ate an average of 2,139 calories, compared to an average of 2,605 in the group eating the lower-protein diet – another testament to the superior appetite-sating potential of protein.

In another study, some individuals were put on a diet containing 17 per cent protein, while others ate a diet containing 23 per cent protein.[8] After six months, the higher-protein group had lost significantly more weight:

8.5 kg compared to 3.9 kg on average. Another trial found that individuals eating a 26 per cent protein diet lost twice as much weight as those eating a 19 per cent protein diet.[9]

In short, there is good evidence that higher-protein diets have distinct advantages for those seeking to lose weight.

WEIGHT LOSS IS ONE THING, FAT LOSS IS ANOTHER

These studies demonstrate the potential for higher-protein diets to promote weight loss. However, as we know, weight loss is one thing, *fat loss* is another. Some studies have looked at fat loss specifically, and the results have been in favour of higher-protein diets.

For example, one of the studies referred to above[10] found that the protein-rich diet led to significantly more fat loss than the one lower in protein (7.6 kg compared to 4.3 kg).

In another study,[11] individuals were tested with diets containing either 1.6 or 0.8 g of protein per kg of body weight. Both diets were calorie-restricted, supplying 500 fewer calories per day than the amount estimated to be required to maintain stable weight. The study lasted for four months.

At the end of the study, those eating the higher-protein diet had lost significantly more fat (8.7 per cent vs 5.7 per cent). Other studies have confirmed the ability of higher-protein diets to yield better results in terms of fat loss.[12, 13]

In another study, a high-protein diet, compared to a high-carb one, led to a significant reduction in waist circumference.[14] Other evidence has found that a higher-protein diet was more effective for shedding abdominal fat in individuals who had a problem in this area.[15]

The evidence suggests that higher-protein diets are effective not just for weight loss, but fat loss specifically, including fat that accumulates around the waist.

PROTEIN AND WEIGHT MAINTENANCE

Many of us have had the experience of losing weight, only to gain it back again (and maybe more) over time. Could more protein in the diet help not just weight loss, but keeping the weight off, too?

In one study, individuals were put on a low-calorie diet for a month.[16] After this, individuals were split into two groups, one of which had their diet supplemented with 30 g of protein each day over a six-month period. The protein-supplemented group regained less than 1 kg in weight, compared to 3 kg in the other group. However, none of the weight regained in the protein-supplemented group came in the form of fat. This was not true for the other group. Higher protein intake was also associated with a reduction in waist circumference, compared to a gain in the other group.

In another study,[17] obese individuals were put on a very low-calorie diet for five to six weeks to induce weight loss. After this, though, individuals were instructed to eat a low-fat diet. Some of the individuals supplemented their diet with carbohydrate (in the form of maltodextrin), while others supplemented their diet with protein (50 g of casein or whey protein each day). Individuals could eat as much of their new diet as they liked for a period of 12 weeks, at which point they were assessed in terms of weight and various biochemical measurements.

At the end of the study, compared to the carb-supplemented individuals, those supplemented with protein lost an average of 2.3 kg more. Crucially, this lost weight was composed almost entirely of *fat*.

Other research had individuals eat either a higher-protein diet (1.6 grams of protein per kg of body weight per day) or lower-protein diet (0.8 grams of protein per kg of body weight per day) for a year.[18] The first four months were designed to provide individuals with a calorie deficit of 500 calories a day, and for the following eight months the calorie intake was designed for weight maintenance (rather than loss).

At the end of the year, while weight loss was not significantly different between the two groups, fat loss was: those on the higher-protein diet did better on this measure. As a group, they had improved body composition (more lean body mass and less fat) compared to those eating the lower-protein diet.

These results suggest that in the longer term, higher-protein diets help individuals to maintain fat loss and are associated with superior body composition.

WHY MIGHT HIGHER-PROTEIN DIETS LEAD TO IMPROVED BODY COMPOSITION?

To improve the body's composition, we can either lose fat, gain muscle, or both. We know that higher-protein diets can be effective for fat loss. Can they help build muscle? Let's start by considering these facts:

1. **Other than water, muscle tissue contains more protein than anything else.**

2. **The building blocks of protein come in the form of what are known as amino acids.**

3. **The body can't make amino acids from carbohydrate or fat – they can only come from protein.**

In other words, to maintain and build muscle, the body requires an adequate intake of protein. Not surprisingly, studies show that higher protein intakes help to retard the loss of muscle that can accompany weight loss.[19] If you're serious about preserving or building muscle, though, appropriate exercise is required. This will be covered in Chapter 10 (Muscle Bound).

So, higher-protein diets do seem to have a lot going for them, in that they can speed fat loss while helping to preserve muscle.

But what about the idea that protein-rich diets can be bad for other aspects of health?

PROTEIN AND THE HEART

Diets rich in protein are sometimes said to have the capacity to induce heart disease. In reality, there is a lot of evidence that higher-protein diets reduce the levels of blood fats known as 'triglycerides'[20,21] which are linked with an increased risk of heart disease.[22] Other evidence links a higher protein intake with a reduced risk of high blood pressure and heart disease.[23] High-protein diets do not appear to pose risks for the heart.

HIGH-PROTEIN DIETS AND THE KIDNEYS

Some doctors and scientists have suggested that high-protein diets may be bad for the kidneys. Yet, two reviews have found no evidence of this in individuals with healthy kidney function.[24,25] In one study, no adverse effects on kidney function tests were detected with protein intakes of up to 2.8 g per kg of body weight per day (that's a lot of protein).[26]

HIGH-PROTEIN DIETS AND BONE HEALTH

Protein is sometimes said to speed the rate at which calcium is lost from the bones, predisposing to weak bones and osteoporosis. Actually, protein is a critical raw material for the manufacture of bone, and higher protein intakes are actually associated with a *reduced* risk of bone fracture.[27,28]

THE PRIMAL PRINCIPLE – PROTEIN

The scientific evidence shows that there are distinct health advantages to eating a high-protein diet. Does this reflect our nutritional past? Analysis reveals that anywhere between 20 and 35 per cent of the calories in primitive hunter-gatherer diets came from protein.[29] In comparison, protein contributes only 16 per cent of calories in the typical UK diet. A protein-rich diet reflects better the diet we evolved on and are best adapted to.

BACK TO BASICS

- Protein is essential for growth and repair in the body, and supplies the raw materials for a wide range of body components including muscle, brain chemicals and the enzymes critical for life itself.

- Eating protein can speed the metabolism to a greater extent than carbohydrate or fat.

- Protein sates the appetite to a greater extent than carbohydrate or fat.

- Higher-protein diets are, compared to lower-protein ones, more effective for the purposes of weight and fat loss.

- Higher-protein diets assist in the maintenance of weight loss.

- Higher-protein diets help to preserve muscle mass during weight loss.

- Higher-protein diets are not inherently hazardous for the health of the kidneys, heart or bone.

Chapter 6

SATISFACTION GUARANTEED

EFFECTIVE STRATEGIES FOR LOSING FAT WITHOUT FEELING FAMISHED

Avoiding the overeating of truly fattening foods is a key component in losing fat and keeping it off. Yet, this can be easier said than done. You may know that the crayfish and avocado salad is the smart choice for lunch, but something in you might be willing you to choose the foot-long baguette instead. Perhaps you can find yourself sometimes yielding to the lure of something sweet in the afternoon. After a substantial dinner, are you irresistibly drawn to a bowl of ice cream or cereal later on? Such episodes not only may sap your resolve, but can also trigger a slide back to the very diet that caused unwanted fatness in the first place.

Another option is just to tough it out and push tempting morsels to one side. The problem here, though, is that you run the risk of consigning yourself to a life of self-restraint and deprivation. Far better, I think, is to manage your eating in a way that neutralises, quite naturally, any tendency to eat more than is required. That is what this chapter is about.

HUNGER IS THE ENEMY

For many seeking to lose weight, hunger is taken as a sure sign that they are in 'calorie deficit' and therefore *must* be losing weight. However, as we explored in Chapter 2 (The Calorie Trap), prolonged under-fuelling of the body can dampen the metabolism, making it more likely that whatever we eat will end up being stored as fat rather than being burned by the body.

Even in the shorter term, though, hunger poses a serious hazard in that it can drive us to eat fat-making carbs, and eat too much of them when we do. Imagine you come home in the evening ravenously hungry. You need something quick and filling. What's it going to be? Some grilled lamb chops with steamed and buttered broccoli and spinach? Probably not. More likely it's going to look like a plateful of pasta or a sandwich. In a restaurant, an overeager appetite could easily cause you to have your fill of complementary bread at the beginning of the meal, and it may well affect your food choices, too. Sitting on a plane or train in a famished state will generally cause us to pile in some pretty disastrous fare.

Now imagine coming to your evening meal in a state where you are ready for food, but not *starving*. In such a state it really is so much easier to do the right thing nutritionally, but without any longing for the not-so-healthy foods you've eschewed.

Not allowing your appetite to run out of control makes healthy eating much easier, whatever the setting.

There are two keys to managing your appetite in a way that makes healthy eating a doddle. They are:

1. **Eating the right food**

2. **Eating it frequently enough.**

Let's take each in turn.

EATING THE RIGHT FOOD

We explored in previous chapters the fact that different foods have different appetite-sating potential. Let's recap on what we've learned so far:

Protein is more sating than the other two major macronutrients. When individuals adopt a higher-protein diet, the tendency is automatically to eat *less* (sometimes a lot less).

The other side to eating a high-protein diet is that it will generally be lower in carbohydrate. This is particularly important when you consider that, as we learned in Chapter 3 (Carb Loading), carbohydrates are not particularly satisfying – this is particularly true for high-GI carbs, which are generally disruptive of blood-sugar levels.

In Chapter 4 (Fat Chance), we saw that fat also has the ability to sate the appetite. This is at least partly related to the fact that it stimulates the secretion of the hormone cholecystokinin, which slows down the rate at which the stomach empties itself and therefore helps prolong feelings of fullness.[1] Studies have found that, for a given number of calories, fat can be more effective at sating the appetite than carbohydrate.[2,3] For some individuals, this appears to be very important indeed. Some men, for instance, will find that a nice fatty piece of lamb or beef or chicken leg will satisfy them much more than, say, a piece of grilled plaice or a skinless chicken breast.

The differing abilities of foods to satisfy the appetite helps to explain how it can be that many of us will find that a handful of nuts (high-protein, high-fat, low GI) will tame an overeager appetite very effectively, while eating a bucket of popcorn (low-protein, low-fat, high-GI) the size of our head will not really touch the sides.

So, in summary, if you want to put a natural brake on your appetite, your diet needs to be high in protein, low in carb, and with enough fat to satisfy you.

EATING THE RIGHT FOOD REGULARLY ENOUGH

Going too long between eating is another major cause of the sort of unbridled hunger that can lead to us making some poor food choices. I can't tell you the number of men (and women) who fall foul of this. Common issues here include skipping breakfast, or alternatively eating something that won't do much to keep hunger at bay such as a croissant, bagel or muesli-style breakfast bar. Not having a half-decent breakfast can leave us so hungry that it becomes almost mandatory to eat a bread-based lunch.

One other frequent issue is the habit some of us have of going too long between lunch and our evening meal. It's not uncommon for eight or more hours to elapse between these meals. This is just too long for most people. If we haven't eaten anything in between, by the time we sit down to dinner, whether at home or not, we can be far too famished to be satisfied by something truly healthy.

Some individuals can safely get away with a bit of infrequency in the feeding department, but such a man is a relatively rare beast in my experience. Three meals a day is the order of the day for most men, and this should be supplemented with healthy snacking when necessary. For the majority, a snack in the late afternoon/early evening will do wonders to keep them on track. Others may require something in the late morning, too.

Details regarding *what* to eat, both at mealtimes and in between, will be laid out in the next chapter.

WON'T ALL THIS EATING MAKE ME FAT?

Deep in the recesses of your psyche, or perhaps on a more conscious level, you may have the belief that all this eating and snacking, even of the 'right' foods, is somehow going to jeopardise your fat-loss efforts. However, it is critical to understand that regular eating can actually lead to less being eaten overall. For example, in one study, the effect of different eating patterns on subsequent eating was tested in a group of overweight men.[4] The study participants were fed a set meal, and five hours later were asked to eat freely from a buffet. At another time, the same men were fed a fifth of the set meal each hour, before being presented with the same food free-for-all. On both occasions, the researchers measured the number of calories consumed at the buffet. Compared to the single meal, the hourly 'snacks' were associated with a reduction in calorie intake at the buffet of more than a quarter.

However, in addition to controlling hunger and making it far easier to eat less (and make healthier choices generally), frequent feeding has other effects that can help you control your weight effectively. For example, consistent eating is associated with reduced levels of insulin – the chief fat-storage hormone in the body.[5,6] It is also linked, perhaps not surprisingly, with increases in metabolism related to the thermogenic effect of food[7] (this phenomenon was discussed in Chapter 5).

Far from being a recipe for weight gain, there are plenty of reasons to believe that regular eating might be a useful tactic for those looking to lose weight. There is even some evidence to support this in the form of a study which showed that the more regularly men ate, the lower their body weight and fatness tended to be.[8] This association even remained after accounting for other factors that might help explain it, such as physical activity and overall food intake. In another study, individuals eating five or more times a day, compared to those eating three or fewer times each day, were half as likely to be overweight.[9]

For optimal weight loss, it looks like it's better to *graze*, than to *gorge*.

GETTING THE BALANCE RIGHT

In Chapter 3 (Carb Loading) we explored how a particular form of hunger may be induced by blood-sugar dropping to sub-normal levels (hypoglycaemia). This tends to trigger an urge for carbohydrate, which can sometimes be overwhelming. When blood-sugar levels are low, it's natural for the body to crave something that will replenish sugar quickly into the bloodstream. Foods of choice tend to be something sweet such as chocolate, biscuits, cakes or sugary soft drinks.

While eating something carb-rich can get us out of a tight spot here, it should be borne in mind that eating a carb-fuelled meal or snack is almost certainly what caused us to arrive in a hypoglycaemic state in the first place. Cutting back on carbs, and putting more emphasis on protein and fat in the diet, really help to stabilize blood-sugar levels, and therefore are key tactics for quelling carb-cravings in time.

If the body has been used to getting ready fuel in the form of fast-releasing carbohydrate, it can take a while for it to adjust to the scaling back of sugar and starch. Some people can end up a bit bereft, which can manifest as carb-cravings that threaten to derail even the most committed of healthy eaters. Should this happen to you, help is at hand ...

CHROMIUM HELPS REDUCE CARB-CRAVINGS

Blood-sugar balance in the body results from physiological and biochemical processes that depend on the supply of key nutrients. Perhaps the most important in this respect is the mineral chromium. And supplementing with chromium does seem to help stabilise blood-sugar levels and, very importantly, can help to curb carb-cravings in particular.

In one study, a group of overweight women were given chromium (1,000 micrograms per day) or placebo (inactive medication) for two months.[10] Compared to women taking the placebo, those taking the chromium supplement saw significantly reduced hunger levels. Food intake was significantly lower for these women, too. In another study, chromium supplementation was found to reduce carbohydrate cravings specifically.[11]

Some supplements offer a blend of nutrients designed to help stabilise blood sugar. In addition to chromium, these often include magnesium and B-vitamins. Such a supplement, or even straight chromium, can be really useful during the initial stages of dietary change, where there can be a tendency for the body to 'miss' the carbs if it has been used to getting plenty of them. Whether in combination with other nutrients or alone, I recommend 400–800 mcg of chromium a day, spread out over 2–3 doses during the day.

GLUTAMINE CAN HELP WITH FOOD CRAVINGS, TOO

Another nutritional agent that can really help quell carb-cravings is the amino acid glutamine. Such cravings are essentially the result of the brain detecting that sugar levels are on the low side. Glutamine provides ready fuel for the brain, and generally quite effectively shuts off cravings, and quickly, too. I suggest buying glutamine as a powder and dissolving 1 teaspoon (about 4 g) in about 500 ml of water. This should be sipped throughout the day, particularly between meals. This is because food cravings are more likely to strike between meals, and also because glutamine is absorbed better when there is not much food in the stomach.

Using chromium-containing supplements and additional glutamine can be highly effective in curbing cravings. Usually such measures are only required for a relatively short period of time while the body adjusts. After two to six weeks it is usually possible to reduce gradually and then stop taking these supplements without any return of troublesome food yearnings.

DARK CHOCOLATE IS THE SWEET TREAT OF CHOICE

For those of us who like to treat ourselves to something sweet and self-indulgent from time to time, my advice is to opt for some dark chocolate (70 per cent cocoa solids or more). One reason for this is that cocoa is actually quite a nutritious substance in its own right, and particularly rich in plant chemicals known as 'polyphenols' that are linked with protection from heart disease. The darker the chocolate, the more cocoa it contains and, importantly, the less sugar. Less sugar means less potential for blood-sugar disruption – and the desire for unhealthy carbs that this can induce.

But there's another reason why dark chocolate is preferred over milk chocolate: people tend to eat less of it. A study from the University of Copenhagen, Denmark in 2008 reported that dark chocolate, gram for gram, is more satisfying than milk chocolate.[12] The higher-protein, lower-GI nature of dark chocolate might have something to do with this.

One other reason for taking a trip to the dark side where chocolate is concerned is that it tends not to have the moreishness of milk chocolate. There's something about the sweetness and texture on the tongue of milk chocolate that means that once people start to eat it, they can find it difficult to stop. This tends not to be the case with dark chocolate, making it a safer option for those seeking a sweet treat without risking derailing their healthy eating regime.

THE APPETITE-DISRUPTERS

Eating the right foods nice and regularly and stabilising blood-sugar levels will go a long way to making sure healthy eating is not a stretch for you. However, it can also be helpful to be aware that certain substances can divert you nonetheless. Specific food additives have the capacity to stimulate the appetite and encourage us to consume calories that are surplus to requirements. The main offenders here are monosodium glutamate (MSG) and artificial sweeteners.

MSG

MSG is a food ingredient which is used to enhance flavour and palatability. MSG (and/or other sources of glutamate) can be found in a wide range of processed foods with the blessing of our governments and food agencies. However, there have been lingering concerns that glutamate might have some adverse affects on health and weight.

MSG is known to have the capacity to stimulate the appetite, which is at least one of the reasons it is used to lace many fast and processed foods. In animals, MSG does not just cause them to eat more,[13] but also stimulates insulin secretion.[14] There is the potential, therefore, that insulin secretion will lead to low blood sugar (hypoglycaemia) some time later, a side effect of which can be ravenous hunger. This might help to explain how it is possible to eat a big Chinese meal (MSG is commonly used in Chinese cuisine) only to find oneself curiously famished just a couple of hours later.

In a study published in the journal *Obesity*, the relationship between MSG consumption and body mass index (BMI) was assessed in a group of individuals aged 40–59.[15] The researchers divided the participants in this study into three bands, according to MSG consumption. Compared to those in the lowest consumption band, those in the highest were found to be 2.75 times more likely to be classified as overweight.

In this study, other than MSG intake, there were no discernable differences in diet or activity levels across the groups. The suggestion here is that glutamate may have one or more metabolic effects in the body which might predispose to weight gain. As it happens, administering MSG to animals has been shown to induce various changes that promote fat accumulation, including the suppression of fat breakdown (lipolysis).[16]

One way to minimise your exposure to glutamate is to scrutinise labels for sources of this substance. They include MSG (obviously), gelatin, hydrolysed vegetable protein (HVP), hydrolysed plant protein, textured protein, autolysed plant protein, yeast extract, autolysed yeast and vegetable protein extract. And this is only a partial list. Of course, if you're having to inspect the ingredients label of a food, you probably haven't got the best food in your hand.

If your diet is made up of ostensibly natural foods like meat, fish, eggs, fruits, vegetables and nuts, then there's not much opportunity for MSG to sneak into your diet. There is little or no need to check labels. Once label-checking is required, then it's likely quite a heavily processed food is being contemplated. A bag of corn chips or packet of soup is rubbish food, whether it's got MSG or any other source of glutamate in it or not. In the next chapter (Sound Bites), we'll be exploring in more depth the virtues of natural, unprocessed foods, as well as the hazards associated with eating more suspect, processed fare.

While you're steering clear of processed foods in supermarkets, give a wide berth to fast food, too, as this is another major provider of MSG and glutamate in the diet.

ARTIFICIAL SWEETENERS

The other major additive appetite-disrupters are artificial sweeteners such as aspartame, sucralose and saccharin. These are generally believed to be better than sugar for those seeking to lose weight on the basis that, while being sweet, they are virtually devoid of calories. However, there is evidence that artificial sweeteners can stimulate the appetite and might actually contribute to weight gain in the long term.

One study, for instance, assessed the effect that artificial sweeteners have on the brain.[17] In this study, women were given a solution containing either the artificial sweetener sucralose (brand name Splenda) or sucrose (table sugar). Brain monitoring showed that sugar activated pleasure centres in the brain more than sucralose.

This difference was found despite the fact that individuals were unable to distinguish between sucrose and sucralose on the basis of taste. In other words, while individuals are unable consciously to distinguish between sugar and sucralose, the brain appears to know the difference. An artificial sweetener may simply not give the level of pleasure and satisfaction that may be derived from sugar. This, in theory, could lead individuals to seek satisfaction from other foodstuffs.

In another study, just putting an artificial sweetener (saccharin) on the tongues of subjects caused insulin levels to rise.[18] As we explored in the section on MSG above, this may induce low blood sugar and the false hunger that can lead to overeating, particularly carbohydrate-rich foodstuffs such as chocolate, biscuits or sweet drinks.

Some evidence shows that artificial sweeteners do indeed have the capacity to stimulate the appetite. For example, one study found that women given saccharin-sweetened lemonade were found to consume considerably more calories overall compared to those drinking regular (sugary) lemonade.[19] In another study, experimenters found that subjects who had eaten yoghurt sweetened with saccharin were inclined to eat more than those who had eaten yoghurt sweetened with sugar.[20] There is other evidence which suggests that aspartame, too, has the capacity to stimulate the appetite.[21]

Animal experiments also call into question the role that artificial sweeteners have in weight control. In one study, rats were fed with either saccharin or sugar-sweetened yoghurt in conjunction with their normal diet.[22] The rats consuming saccharin ate more calories than their sugar-eating counterparts. Not only this, but they gained more weight, and more *fat*, too. The authors of this study concluded that '... using artificial sweeteners in rats resulted in increased caloric intake, increased body weight, and increased adiposity', and that 'These results suggest that consumption of products containing artificial sweeteners may lead to increased body weight and obesity by interfering with fundamental homeostatic, physiological processes.' Chapter 8 (Liquid

Assets) includes information about other health hazards associated with consuming artificial sweeteners.

There is no good scientific evidence that artificial sweeteners aid weight loss. If anything, the reverse is true.

CAN SALT MAKE YOU FAT?

Salt – sodium chloride for the chemically inclined – is sprinkled liberally in the Western diet. About 90 per cent of the salt we consume comes as part and parcel of processed foods, including ready meals and fast food. However, even seemingly innocuous foods can contain a stack of salt. Did you know that cornflakes, weight for weight, have the same salt content as sea water?

Salt is well known for its ability to raise blood pressure, which can up the risk of 'cardiovascular' diseases, particularly stroke. But could salt somehow contribute to weight gain, too?

One mechanism that may be at play relates to the fact that salty foods can make us thirsty. Now, if all we drink is pure, unadulterated H_2O, then that's one thing (though some fluid retention may occur as a result). But if our drinks of choice happen to be sugary tea, coffee, soft drinks or beer, then problems may ensue.

The effect of salt consumption and foodstuff consumption has not been formally assessed in adults, but it has in children and adolescents. In one study, it was found that as salt intake increased, so did fluid intake.[23] In fact, for each additional gram of salt consumed each day, fluid intake increased by about 100 g per day. About half of the subjects' total fluid intake was in the form of soft drinks.

The authors of this study estimated that if childhood salt consumption was halved (from about 6 g to 3 g per day), then this would lead to an average reduction of about 2.5 sugary soft drinks per week per child. Part of the relevance of this relates to the fact that there is quite a lot of evidence out there now that sugar-sweetened drinks are a potential driver of weight gain and obesity. The same, of course, is true of sugar-charged beverages or alcohol in the adult world.

Most of us will have had the experience of going into a bar and finding complimentary savoury snacks to nibble on as we drink, such as crisps, salted peanuts, pretzels and Japanese rice crackers. In the past you may have been tempted to resist the urge to eat them on the basis that they may well be laced with other people's urine. Now you have another reason not to eat them: salt, and its tendency to cause you to drink more than you otherwise would.

SPEED-EATING CAN LEAD TO OVEREATING

You probably won't find the fact that the hungrier we are, the quicker we tend to eat much of a revelation. However, the important thing is that the faster we eat, the *more* we may end up eating before the brain tells us that we've had enough. An overeager appetite and 'express eating' could, therefore, predispose to excess weight. In a study published in the *British Medical Journal* it was found that rapid-eating men, compared to slower-eating ones, were almost twice as likely to be overweight.[24]

The question is: could slowing down and chewing food more thoroughly help to prevent overeating? It seems so.

In one study, 30 women were asked to eat a pasta-based meal under two distinct conditions.[25] At one sitting, they were asked to take small bites and chew each one 15–20 times. At another sitting, they were asked to eat as quickly as possible. The women were also instructed to eat until they were satisfied.

Compared to the rapid eaters, the women instructed to take their time and chew thoroughly consumed about 70 fewer calories. Not only that, but these women felt more satisfied immediately after the meal and an hour later.

This study suggests that getting too hungry, and the speed-eating this can induce, could quite easily cause us to eat food that is surplus to requirements.

Other evidence for the importance of slowing food intake down has come in the form of a study published in the *American Journal of Clinical Nutrition*.[26] Here, a group were given semi-solid chocolate custard to eat under a number of different circumstances. For example, in one test, individuals were instructed to consume the custard using relatively small bites (5 grams of custard in each bite). At another time, they were instructed to take larger bites (15 grams). In both of these settings, test subjects were also asked to process the food in their mouths quickly (3 seconds before swallowing) and slowly (9 seconds per bite). In all test settings, individuals were instructed to eat as much as they wanted and to stop when pleasantly satisfied.

One notable finding from this study was that less was eaten when the subjects took small bites compared to large bites. Average intake was about 100 fewer calories (about a 23 per cent calorie reduction). Also, though, the longer the oral processing time, the less was eaten, too (longer processing time was associated with a reduced intake in the order of 70 calories for small bite sizes and 50 calories for larger bite sizes).

The results of this study suggest that taking small bites and chewing them thoroughly (to increase oral processing time) may lead to a natural reduction in the amount of food consumed during a meal.

It is also worth bearing in mind that there is other evidence which supports the concept that what happens in the mouth can have a bearing on the satisfaction derived from food and how much of it is eaten. Research has found that food is more satisfying if it's actually eaten rather than just infused into the gut through a tube. Taking time to savour food properly may help us get more enjoyment from less food.

HERE COMES THE 'CHEW-CHEW' – TIPS FOR SLOWER EATING

1. **Avoid getting too hungry before meals**
   This is the most important thing of all – it's very difficult to eat in a controlled fashion and savour food if you're ravenous. A higher-protein, lower-carb diet will help here, but use of healthy snacking can play a part, too. Eating something (e.g. nuts) in the late afternoon or early evening is, for most men, a necessary step in controlling appetite at the end of the day.

2. **Put less on your fork or spoon**
   Be conscious of how much food you're putting into your mouth. If you're stacking your fork or piling your spoon high with food, you might want to rethink this. Make a conscious effort to keep each mouthful small and manageable.

3. **Chew thoroughly**
   Thorough chewing aids digestion, and also slows down the eating process. Make a conscious effort to chew each mouthful of food 20 times before swallowing.

While you are chewing, perhaps put your cutlery down, and don't pick it up again until you've fully chewed and swallowed the last mouthful.

4. Eat mindfully

Sometimes our eating can be driven not just by hunger and food preferences, but other factors such as boredom, stress and habit. Eating 'mindfully' can help, and practical suggestions regarding this are covered in the final chapter (Mind Matters).

SHOP WITHOUT HUNGER

In this chapter the importance of not getting too hungry before eating has been emphasised. This same approach should be applied to food shopping, too. Going around the supermarket or convenience store in a ravenous state is just asking for trouble. The best time to go food shopping is after a meal or substantial snack. Having a satisfied stomach makes putting exclusively healthy foods in your basket far easier.

BACK TO BASICS

- Ensuring that we are well satisfied by food is a key to sustainable fat loss.

- For the diet to be satisfying, it generally needs to be relatively rich in protein and low in carbohydrate.

- Regular meals, and possibly snacks, are important for regulating appetite and food intake.

- Regular eating is associated with physiological benefits, including lower insulin levels and improved enhancement of the metabolism through the thermogenic effect of food.

- Episodes of low blood sugar (hypoglycaemia) can stimulate hunger and, in particular, cravings for carbohydrate.

- Chromium, and other nutrients including magnesium and certain B-vitamins, can help stabilise blood-sugar levels and combat food cravings.

- The amino acid glutamine provides ready fuel for the brain and can be effective in combating food cravings, too.

- MSG and other sources of glutamate can stimulate the appetite and should be avoided.

- Artificial sweeteners, similarly, can disrupt the appetite and may predispose to weight gain.

- Eating slowly, chewing thoroughly and savouring food can all help prevent overeating.

- Avoid food shopping when hungry.

Chapter 7

SOUND BITES

WHAT TO EAT FOR FAST FAT LOSS AND OPTIMAL HEALTH

Previously in this book we have examined the impact of different types of foodstuffs on body weight, body composition and general health. We've also explored food from a hunger perspective, and in particular which foods are most likely to sate our appetite and prevent overeating.

In this chapter we're going to take this theory and apply it to real foods in the real world. Specific foods will be judged on the basis of what we've learned so far, as well as other important nutritional criteria (outlined below). Let's recap, first, on the qualities we're looking for in the foods we eat.

1. **Protein**
   Higher-protein foods are generally preferred to lower-protein foods. Protein-rich diets help weight and fat loss, at least partly because of the fact that, calorie for calorie, protein sates the appetite more than carbohydrate or fat. Protein is also essential for the building and maintenance of muscle and a healthy body composition.

2. Carbohydrate

Certain carbohydrates tend to disrupt blood-sugar and insulin levels in a way that predisposes to fatty accumulation in the body. Foods that pose the most hazards in this respect are those of the highest glycaemic index/load (principally starch and foods with added sugar). These foods also tend to have limited appetite-sating potential, and may even stimulate hunger and carbohydrate cravings through their ability to induce blood-sugar lows (hypoglycaemia). In addition to their disruptive effects on blood sugar and insulin, many of these foods have little to offer from a nutritional perspective. Better sources of carbohydrate will be those that are not disruptive to blood sugar and insulin, and are more nutritious, too (principally, fruits and vegetables).

3. Fat

Fats occurring naturally in the diet do not appear to be fattening, nor do they appear to have adverse effects on health. Fats that appear to be positively beneficial to health include monounsaturated and omega-3 fats. Foods rich in these fats should be emphasized in the diet. Industrially produced partially-hydrogenated and trans fats, which are linked with an increased risk of heart disease and other adverse effects on health, should be avoided. Foods rich in omega-6 fats should be used sparingly.

4. Additives

Artificial additives should be avoided, especially MSG and artificial sweeteners, as these have the ability to disrupt appetite control and stimulate hunger.

There are some other dietary components that demand consideration when assessing foods, including micro-nutrients, phytochemicals and fibre.

5. **Micronutrients (vitamins and minerals)**
Foods rich in micronutrients should be emphasised in the diet.

6. **Phytochemicals**
Phytochemicals are plant-derived substances which have health-promoting and disease-protective properties. Foods rich in phytochemicals (e.g. fruits and vegetables) should be emphasised in the diet.

7. **Fibre**
Fibre comes in two main forms: soluble and insoluble. Insoluble fibre (found in foods such as wholegrain wheat and bran) is often recommended for bowel health, though studies suggest that it has limited benefit here. On the other hand, soluble fibre tends to improve bowel symptoms.[1] It is found in foods such as fruits, vegetables, nuts and seeds.

Those are the rules. Let's see how specific foods measure up when we apply them.

Any positive and negative features of each major foodstuff will be highlighted. The food will also be given an overall rating regarding whether it is to be eaten freely, in moderation, or not at all. These ratings are summarised in a table at the end of this chapter.

WHAT DOES 'MODERATION' MEAN?

Some of the foods here are recommended 'in moderation'. But what does *moderation* mean? What it means, in essence, is that wherever possible, opt for foods that are earmarked for unlimited eating. However, when it becomes difficult to eat from free foods, or you just fancy something else, quite frankly it's OK to eat something from the 'in moderation' list.

Here's how this may work in practice. Let's imagine your two main meals of the day are generally made up of meat or fish with salad or vegetables from the 'eat freely' category. One night you cook some sausages and decide that some Puy lentils (an 'in moderation' food) would go well with them. There's no need to hold back here, but do aim to make including such a food in meals the exception and not the rule. At the same time you might like to accompany the lentils with something from the 'unlimited' list (e.g. cabbage or broccoli) so that the lentils assume less prominence in the meal.

In the early stages of adjusting your diet, I recommend having a modest portion of an 'in moderation' food no more than once a day. However, once you are close to or have achieved your health goals, you can relax this. Even when you do, however, it is important to aim to ensure that the bulk (about 80 per cent) of your diet is made up of the 'eat freely' foods.

MEAT

Meat is a high-protein, low-carb food, and ideal for individuals wanting to lose fat and build muscle. The saturated fat in meat has not been shown to pose hazards for health (see Chapter 5 – Fat Chance). It's also worth bearing in mind that about half the fat in meats such as lamb and beef is monounsaturated (heart-healthy) in nature.

Meat is rich in certain micronutrients, too, including iron (important for energy production and an essential component of the haemoglobin in red blood cells, which carries oxygen around the body) and zinc (which plays an important role in, amongst other things, immune function, wound-healing ability, brain function and fertility). As far as vitamins are concerned, meat offers a rich complement of B-vitamins, including B_1 (thiamin), B_2 (riboflavin), B_3 (niacin), B_6 and B_{12}. These nutrients have a wide range of functions in the body, and assist both in the generation of energy and in balanced brain function.

Another of meat's nutritional offerings comes in the form of carnitine – a substance comprised of two amino acids: lysine and methionine. One of carnitine's chief roles is to help the conversion of fat into energy in the body's cells. Meat is also rich in the amino acid leucine, which studies show helps to prevent muscle loss during weight loss.[2]

Meat Quality

Many commercially reared animals are intensively farmed, and often exposed to drugs and chemicals that taint their meat. These may have undesirable effects when subsequently consumed by humans. One of the worst meats in this respect is chicken. While poultry is generally regarded as healthier than 'red' meats such as beef and lamb, this is not necessarily the case. Most chickens are kept in miserable conditions and loaded with growth-promoting antibiotics during their brief lives.

Chicken is one meat almost certainly worth eating in its organic, free-range form. The same is also true of pork, which is another usually intensively reared meat. Going organic is probably the best option for other meats such as lamb and beef, though this is generally less of a concern here as these animals, particularly sheep, are generally less intensively reared. Other options include game meats such as venison, partridge, pheasant and duck.

Also, there is evidence that the type of feed animals eat during their lives has a bearing on the nutritional profile of the meat they produce. Animals such as cows and sheep are adapted, essentially, to eating grass. Yet in the intensive rearing of animals, grass is often substituted with grain. Compared to grain-fed animals, those which have been grass-fed end up having high levels of the so-called omega-3 fats, which have been associated with a range of benefits for body and brain.[3]

The processing of meat is another potential concern. There is a world of difference between an unadulterated organic chicken breast and a chicken nugget. The latter is likely to contain poor quality meat and a range of additives. Also, processed meats such as bacon, sausage and salami generally contain preservative chemicals such as sodium nitrite, which has links with stomach cancer[4] and brain tumours.[5]

DOES RED MEAT CAUSE COLON CANCER?

One form of cancer that is often said to be related to meat-eating, particularly red meat, is colon cancer. In one review, both red and processed meat were found to be associated with this condition.[6] One of the problems with this review, however, is that it did not take into account other factors related to colon cancer such as, say, vegetable consumption. Someone eating lots of meat might be at increased risk of colon cancer, not because of all the red meat he's eating, but because of the relative lack of vegetables in the diet. Studies that do not take into account these so-called 'confounding factors' are therefore quite unreliable for determining links between diet and disease.

Another review found that of 44 relevant studies, most (31) found no apparent association between red meat intake and colon cancer risk.[7] This review suggested that any heightened risk of colon cancer comes mainly from eating processed meats. Some more evidence for the proposed role of processed foods in colon cancer came from a study published in the *International Journal of Cancer*, which found that, weight for weight, processed meat has significantly more cancer-causing potential in the colon than red meat.[8]

With the evidence as it stands, it makes sense that if we're going to eat meat, then this should come predominantly from animals reared as naturally as possible. And, as a general rule, meat should be eaten in unprocessed form. Hunks of meat like steak, lamb and chicken are, generally speaking, to be preferred to foods such as sausages, ham, bacon and salami.

Another step in the right direction with regard to meat is to buy it in a farm shop, farmers' market or butcher shop, where the origin of the animal is more likely to be assured. Using your purchasing power in these places may also help to support the local economy.

Summary

- **Meat can be eaten freely (organic and/or naturally reared meat is preferred).**

- **Processed meats should be eaten in moderation.**

FISH AND SEAFOOD

Fish and seafood (such as prawns, crab, mussels) are both rich in protein and low in carbohydrate. Like meat, they are good foods to be eaten by individuals seeking to lose fat.

Fish and seafood also tend to be good sources of zinc (see section on Meat, above, for some of the benefits this nutrient brings to the body). They are also rich in iodine, which is vitally important for the proper functioning of the thyroid gland, which itself has a vital role to play in regulating metabolism and health in general. One other common constituent of seafood and fish is vitamin D, which, among other things, plays a part in bone and muscle health. Mounting evidence links higher levels of vitamin D with a reduced risk of cancer, cardiovascular disease, diabetes and premature death.

Some forms of fish, notably salmon, mackerel, trout, sardines and herring, are very rich in omega-3 fats.

However, as with meat, some questions have been raised about potential contaminants to be found in fish. Mercury, for instance, is a potential contaminant in fish such as tuna, marlin and swordfish, and has the potential to cause neurological damage. Fish, particularly farmed fish, may be contaminated with substances such as dioxins and polychlorinated biphenyls (PCBs), which are believed to have cancer-promoting effects in the body. Happily, when the overall impact of fish-eating on health was assessed, the conclusion was that it does more good than harm.[9]

Another potential cause for concern is the depleted fish stocks in our seas. As a result, fish-farming is now increasingly being used to meet demand (and generally at a lower price, too). Fish farming generally involves exposing fish to chemicals (such as antibiotics and colourings) that are not encountered in the wild. Also, fish farming is bad news from an ecological perspective.

In an ideal world, fish is best consumed in wild rather than farmed form. However, fresh fish is generally expensive, and we need to be mindful of the depleted fish stocks in our seas. For a guide to the best fish to eat from a sustainability and ecological point of view, see http://www.fishonline.org.

Canned fish, though not as good as fresh from a nutritional perspective, can offer a more cost-effective way of consuming fish. The most popular canned fish in the UK is tuna. Tuna is often referred to as an 'oily' fish. However, while fresh tuna does contain some omega-3 (though not nearly as much as fish such as salmon and mackerel), much of this is removed before canning. Tuna is also one of the fish, along with marlin and swordfish, that tends to be contaminated with mercury (see above). This does not mean that such fish needs be avoided altogether. However, better types of fish to have from a can are salmon, mackerel and sardines: these are richer in omega-3 fatty acids, and tend not to be contaminated with mercury.

Summary

- **Fresh fish and seafood are foods to be eaten freely.**

- **Tuna, marlin and swordfish are to be eaten in moderation.**

- **Canned fish, besides tuna, can be eaten freely.**

IS A VEGETARIAN DIET INHERENTLY HEALTHY?

There is a general view that vegetarian diets are healthier than more omnivorous ones. Proponents of vegetarianism on health grounds often point to studies which show vegetarians to have a lower risk of heart disease and even overall risk of death. However, such studies are what are known as 'epidemiological' in nature, which means that while they can show *associations* between two factors (in this case, vegetarian eating and better health), these studies cannot be used to *prove* that vegetarianism is healthy.

The reason for this is that the apparent benefits to health may come from other factors associated with vegetarianism, such as a reduced tendency to smoke, and healthier exercise habits, rather than the absence of meat and fish in the diet. These so-called 'confounding factors' need to be taken into consideration in order to make a fair assessment of the relative merits of vegetarian and non-vegetarian diets.

There are now several studies which have attempted to 'level the playing field' when comparing the health of vegetarians and non-vegetarians. In one study, researchers attempted to counteract confounding factors by focusing only on individuals who shopped in health food stores.[10] The idea here was that all of these individuals were similarly 'health-conscious', whether they were vegetarian or not. This allows a fairer appraisal of the impact of vegetarian or non-vegetarian eating. Overall risk of death (the broadest and best measure of health) was not different between vegetarians and non-vegetarians.

In another study, vegetarians were asked to recruit their friends and family into the study. Doing this was thought to help ensure that all individuals in the study were, again, similarly health-conscious. As with the previous study, death rates for vegetarians and non-vegetarians were the same.[11] Other research looked at total mortality in a large group of vegetarians and non-vegetarians.[12] Confounding factors such as age, sex, smoking and alcohol consumption were taken into account in the analysis. The result? No difference in the risk of death between vegetarians and non-vegetarians.

The results of these studies show that vegetarian diets do not have broad health benefits compared to those containing meat and/or fish.

EGGS

Eggs, like meat, fish and seafood, are rich in protein and low in carbohydrate. This makes them a good food for individuals seeking to lose fat and/or build muscle.

Eggs, along with red meat, have generally been caught up in the anti-fat hysteria that most of us will be familiar with. However, we know saturated fat and cholesterol are not to be feared. Besides, the most plentiful type of fat to be found in eggs is actually of the monounsaturated variety – a type of fat associated with a reduced risk of heart disease.

Other nutrients supplied by eggs include B vitamins (especially vitamins B_2 and B_{12}), as well as vitamins A and D.

There are studies in the scientific literature which have linked egg-eating and heart disease. Such studies are 'epidemiological' in nature, and many of them have failed to take into account confounding factors. The most recent comprehensive review of the relationship between specific foodstuffs and heart disease risk found that eating eggs is not associated with an increased risk of this condition.[13]

Summary

- **Eggs can be eaten freely.**

FRUIT

Fruits are generally nutritious foods offering, for example, relatively high levels of micronutrients (including vitamin C) as well as soluble fibre. Fruits are also rich in phytochemicals. For example, citrus fruits and apples are rich in hesperidin and flavonols respectively (both of these phytochemicals are linked with a reduced risk of heart disease), while strawberries and other berries offer a phytochemical by the name of ellagic acid (which appears to have significant cancer-protective properties).

One potential problem with fruit is the fact that it is generally very rich in carbohydrate – specifically sugar in the form of fructose (see Chapter 3 for more about this). To my mind, though, there is no comparison between eating an apple and eating a doughnut. Although both contain quite a lot of sugar, one of these foods is actually very nutritious and releases its sugar quite slowly into the bloodstream, while the other is nutritionally bereft, releases sugar quite quickly, and is likely to be laced with unhealthy fats, too. Also, generally speaking, fruit contains less sugar than foods with added sugar. Nonetheless, the high-sugar nature of many fruits means they are not necessarily something to emphasise in the diet if fat loss and optimum health are the goal.

Probably the best fruits are berries, as these are relatively low in sugar and also offer a great deal in terms of nutrient content. Avocado pears are another good choice, chiefly because they are relatively protein-packed and fat-rich compared to other fruits. Other fruits, such as apples, pears, peaches, nectarines, plums and citrus fruits, should be eaten in moderation. Certain tropical fruits, including banana, mango and pineapple, are quite carb-rich and are best eaten in quite limited quantities until your weight and health goals are met. Dried fruit is intensely sugary, and should be avoided except in small quantities.

Summary

- **Berries and avocado can be eaten freely.**

- **All other fresh fruits can be eaten in moderation.**

- **Dried fruit should be eaten in small quantities only.**

FRUIT, VEGETABLES AND AGROCHEMICALS

Whilst fruits and vegetables should assume a generally prominent place in our diet, there is always the potential that they will come laced with unwanted chemicals. A lot of fresh produce is quite liberally treated with agrochemicals such as pesticides and fungicides, designed to keep it free from attack by insects and moulds. These chemicals are designed to kill things, and common sense dictates that the fewer of these chemicals we consume, the better.

With this in mind, fruit and vegetables are still almost certainly a healthier option than regular fare. While organic produce is the best choice for a number of reasons, its often premium price can put it beyond the reach of many. Very thorough washing of fresh produce will at least help to reduce the negative impact pesticide residues may have on health.

VEGETABLES

Vegetables that grow above the ground, such as broccoli, cabbage, cauliflower and kale, are low in carbohydrate and, coupled with the fact that they are generally highly nutritious (rich in, for example, folate, vitamin C, phytochemicals and soluble fibre), are highly recommended foods.

Vegetables that grow below the ground, such as carrots, parsnips, swede and sweet potato, are richer in carbohydrate and should be eaten in moderation. Squash and pumpkin are also relatively carb-rich, and should be eaten in moderation. Onion, even though it grows beneath ground, is relatively low in carb and can be eaten freely. White potatoes (see below) should be avoided.

THE POTATO – A VEGETABLE IN A CLASS OF ITS OWN

Vegetables are generally healthy for all types of people, but one exception is the potato. Unlike most other vegetables, the potato has a relatively high glycaemic index and load. It is also a vegetable that tends to offer little in the way of nutritional value compared to other vegetables such as leafy greens. For these reasons, white potatoes are not recommended.

This does not mean that they should not be eaten at all. It does mean, however, that they should not take prominence in a meal (e.g. a huge baked potato). I advise using them sparingly (e.g. a little potato in a casserole, or a few new potatoes alongside some meat or fish and vegetables) or not at all.

Summary

- Green and leafy vegetables can be eaten freely, as can onions.

- Squash, pumpkin, sweet potato, carrots, swede and parsnips should be eaten in moderation.

- Potato should be avoided except in very limited quantities.

BEANS AND LENTILS

Beans and lentils are collectively referred to as pulses or 'legumes'. This class of foods also includes peas and peanuts. Legumes are a relatively recent addition to the human diet (about 10,000 years ago). Legumes have some capacity to trigger unwanted food-sensitivity reactions. The food components in legumes which may be responsible for these unwanted reactions are called lectins. Legumes also contain substances that impair the action of digestive enzymes in the gut, such as amylase and trypsin.[14] These 'enzyme inhibitors' impair the digestion of food, which can increase the risk of food sensitivity and may reduce the nutritional value that can be derived from food, too.

On the plus side, there is evidence that the lectins and enzyme inhibitors found in legumes can be at least partially deactivated by thorough soaking and cooking (see below).

The inherent problems legumes pose need to be weighed against the fact that they are a reasonably nutritious food. Peas, peanuts and most beans and lentils are eaten 'whole' – something that is in stark contrast to the refined, nutrient-stripped form we find in so many grains within our diet. Also – again, unlike many grains – legumes generally have low GIs and GLs, which has important implications for health and wellbeing (see Chapter 3 for more details about this).

In one study, the relationship between different types of foods and longevity was assessed in Japan, Sweden, Greece and Australia.[15] Of all the food analysed, the only one that was consistently associated with increased lifespan was legumes. This does not, of course, prove that legumes were the life-extending factor. But the results of this study at least support the notion that beans and lentils have some place in a healthy diet.

Pulses can be used as an accompaniment to a meal (e.g. peas or Puy lentils), or as an addition to salads, stews or soups. Home-made hummus, the main ingredient of which is chickpeas, is another option. Baked beans, on account of their high sugar and salt content, should be regarded as nutritionally inferior to less processed forms of pulses and are not recommended.

PREPARING PULSES

Legumes can contain substances called lectins which may be responsible for food-sensitivity reactions, as well as 'enzyme inhibitors' that can impair digestion. These components can be deactivated, to a large degree, by preparing and cooking pulses properly.

As far as preparation is concerned, soaking is the key. If you intend cooking beans from their dried state, they should first be soaked for several hours (generally 4–12 hours). The most convenient time to do this is generally overnight. The soaking water should then be discarded, and the beans should be rinsed before cooking in unsalted water (salt tends to toughen their skins).

An alternative to this lengthy preparation time is to buy canned pulses. However, before preparation, rinse them thoroughly as this will help to remove as much added salt and sugar as possible.

Thorough cooking of legumes will not just help to nullify lectins and enzyme inhibitors, but can also reduce the levels of certain starches in beans that can ferment in the gut and cause wind.[16]

Summary

• **Legumes should be eaten in moderation.**

SOYA

Perhaps one of the most widely eaten beans of all is the soybean. Actually, the bean itself is hardly, if ever, eaten, but food products prepared from components of the bean are. The oil derived from soybeans finds its way into many processed foods. Also, the protein-rich part of the bean can be used as the basis for a wide range of foods including tofu, soya milk, tempeh and miso. There have been a range of health claims made for soy, including an ability to reduce cholesterol levels and ward off breast cancer and osteoporosis. Actually, though, the evidence suggests that soy is not the versatile wonderfood it is so often made out to be.

First of all, despite its widespread use in the diet, soya is actually a relatively new food – soybeans were probably first cultivated no more than 3,000 years ago. Like other legumes, soybeans contain substances that can impair digestion, which in turn can reduce the nutritional value of the foods we eat and enhance the risk of food sensitivities, too. Although these toxic compounds are largely deactivated or removed during the processing of soybeans into products such as tofu, tempeh and miso, there is the risk that at least some of them will remain in the finished product, thus having implications for health.

Soybeans are also rich in a substance known as phytic acid – a compound which impairs the absorption of a range of minerals including calcium, magnesium, iron and zinc. Phytic acid is also found in grains, but soybeans seem to be especially rich in this anti-nutrient.[17] Unfortunately, cooking does not seem to destroy phytic acid, though levels of this compound can be reduced (though not necessarily eliminated) by fermentation to make foods such as tempeh and miso.

The processing of soya involves converting the soybeans into something known as soy protein isolate (SPI). Production of SPI takes place in factories where a slurry of soybeans is treated with acid and alkali solutions to get the protein to precipitate out. In this process the product can be tainted with the metal aluminium (aluminium exposure has been linked with an increased risk of degeneration of the nervous system and Alzheimer's disease). The resultant protein-rich 'curd' is spray-dried at high temperature to produce a powder. SPI may then be heated and extruded under pressure to make a foodstuff known as textured vegetable protein (TVP). SPI and TVP will often have monosodium glutamate (MSG) added to it to impart a 'meaty' flavour (see Chapter 6 for details on why MSG should be avoided). Once flavoured, SPI can be shaped into a wide range of foods including meat-substitute products such as vegetarian burgers, sausages and mince.

Versatile SPI may be, but it is actually a very heavily processed food. What are its effects on health? Certain toxins found in soya, including digestion inhibitors, are known to remain in SPI.[18] Animal experiments suggest that eating SPI can lead to a deficiency in a range of nutrients including calcium, magnesium, manganese, copper, iron and zinc.[19] Soy also seems to have the capacity to impair thyroid function, which can lead to diverse symptoms such as weight gain, fatigue and constipation.[20]

Soya has been shown to reduce cholesterol levels – though, as we learned in Chapter 4, this does not have broad benefits for health. Soya has also been heavily promoted for its breast-cancer-protective effects. This proposed benefit has been put down to hormone-like molecules known as phytoestrogens, found in soya. These are often said to help block the breast-cancer-causing potential of the hormone oestrogen in the female body. However, the evidence in this area is very mixed, and there is simply no clear evidence which supports the role of dietary phytoestrogens in preventing breast cancer.[21]

Also, it is possible that plant compounds which mimic oestrogen may actually have an adverse effect on health. It is known, for instance, that high levels of oestrogen have been associated with an increased rate of mental decline associated with ageing. One study has found a significant statistical relationship between eating tofu and accelerated brain ageing.[22] As a man, you may be interested to know that higher soya intake has been associated with lower semen quality.[23]

Finally, soy contains substances that can impair the function of the thyroid and thyroid hormones, something which can have profound implications for weight and health. Feeding rats a constituent in soya known as genistein has been found to cause irreversible damage to the enzymes that make thyroid hormones in the body.[24]

The balance of evidence suggests that soy-based foods are not to be emphasised in the diet. Forms of soy that seem particularly worth avoiding are SPI and TVP. The best forms of soy are likely to be more natural forms of this food which have also been fermented, such as tempeh, natto and miso.

Summary

- **Soya-based foods should be avoided, other than tempeh, natto and miso, which may be eaten in moderation.**

QUORN

Another food favourite of vegetarians, vegans or individuals just wanting to eat more 'healthily' is Quorn. The main ingredient in this foodstuff is 'mycoprotein'. Mycoprotein actually comes from a mould organism (*Fusarium venenatum*) that was discovered in soil samples by British scientists in the 1960s. This organism is then multiplied en masse in steel containers and then contrived into foods such as burgers, sausages and meat.

Quorn's manufacturers like to give its product a natural

'flavour' by likening it to mushrooms and truffles. However, according to Professor David Geiser of the Fusarium Research Center at Pennsylvania State University in the USA, drawing parallels between the organism used to make Quorn and mushrooms is like 'calling a rat a chicken because both are animals'.[25] Perhaps not surprisingly, this novel food has been linked with adverse reactions including gastrointestinal complaints.[26]

Like SPI and TVP (see Soy, above), Quorn is a highly processed and quite unnatural food of dubious nutritional merit.

Summary

- **Quorn should be avoided.**

NUTS AND SEEDS

Tree nuts such as walnuts, pecans, cashews, hazelnuts and almonds are relatively protein-rich, low-carb foods. Nuts are very fatty and calorific, but as we discovered in Chapter 4 (Fat Chance), they are not fattening and may actually assist with weight loss. It should also be borne in mind that, while about 80 per cent of the calories nuts offer come from fat, much of this can come in the so-called monounsaturated form believed to have benefits for the heart and circulation.

Nuts are also rich in nutrients such as magnesium, potassium, copper and vitamin E – all of which may benefit cardiovascular health. Nut eating is associated with a reduced risk of heart disease. One study found that women consuming at least five ounces (about 125 g) of nuts each week had one-third fewer heart attacks compared to women who rarely or never ate nuts.[27] In another study, men eating nuts twice a week, compared to those who rarely or never ate nuts, were found to be at about half the risk of a condition known as 'sudden cardiac death'.[28]

Seeds (e.g. pumpkin, sesame, sunflower) have not been formally studied with regard to their effects on health. Because they are nutritionally very similar to nuts, however, we would expect them to have broadly similar benefits for the heart.

Nuts are best eaten in their most unadulterated form – raw. However, they can also be eaten roasted and salted, as long as you do not have a history of raised blood pressure.

Summary

- **Nuts and seeds can be eaten freely and should preferably be eaten in their raw form.**

COOKING OILS

Many vegetable oils, such as sunflower, soya and corn oils, are rich in omega-6 fats, a general excess of which are in the diet. Healthier options include olive oil and avocado oil (both rich in monounsaturated fat) and coconut oil (rich in saturated fat). Sesame oil contains roughly equal amounts of omega-6 and monounsaturated fat, and may be used in moderation.

Summary

- **Olive oil, avocado oil, and coconut oil may be eaten freely.**

- **Sesame oil may be eaten in moderation.**

- **Other vegetable oils should be avoided.**

BUTTER AND MARGARINE

The bulk of butter comes from saturated and monounsaturated fats – two fats that have been in the human diet forever. As we discovered in Chapter 4, saturated fat does not appear to have adverse effects on health, and monounsaturated fat appears to be heart-healthy. Fat does not stimulate insulin secretion, and therefore does not in and of itself cause fat accumulation in the body.

Butter is good as an addition to cooked vegetables (e.g. spinach, asparagus, carrots) or scrambled eggs.

Margarine is a highly processed, chemicalised food that appears to have adverse effects on health (see Chapter 4 for more on this).

Summary

- **Butter can be eaten freely.**

- **Margarine should be avoided.**

DAIRY PRODUCTS

Other than butter (see above), the main dairy products are milk, cheese, yoghurt, cream and ice cream.

One potential effect that food has in the body is something known as food 'sensitivity' (also known as food 'intolerance'). Here, the body can react adversely to a food, giving rise to symptoms which may include digestive discomfort and wind, asthma, eczema, nasal/sinus congestion, mucus/catarrh and fatigue.

One commonly recognised problem with dairy products relates to the sugar (lactose) they can contain. An inability to digest this sugar, called lactose intolerance, affects the majority of the world's population (principally non-Caucasians). Lactose intolerance tends to cause gut-related symptoms such as bloating, wind and diarrhoea.

The other major element that appears to have the capacity to trigger unwanted reactions are proteins in dairy products, such as casein. The theory here is that we are simply not well adapted to these proteins, don't digest them well, and can therefore leak them through the gut wall into the bloodstream, where they can trigger unwanted reactions. Critical to this issue seems to be the processing of pasteurisation. My experience in practice is that many individuals can tolerate raw dairy products, but react to those that have been pasteurised. Part of the explanation for this may lie in the fact that pasteurisation can change the protein molecules in dairy products in a way that makes them harder to digest, and will therefore make them more likely to trigger unwanted symptoms.

Milk is rich in lactose and casein and, as dairy products go, is generally the most problematic from a food-sensitivity perspective. Its relatively high sugar content is another reason to avoid it.

In practice, yoghurt is better tolerated than milk. Studies show that the bacteria deployed in the fermentation process that converts milk into yoghurt aid the digestion of milk proteins.[29,30] The pre-digestion of protein by bacteria helps to explain why, compared to milk, yoghurt is less likely to provoke food-sensitivity reactions.

An added benefit is that some strains of bacteria used in making yoghurt have lactose-digesting ability; this is reflected in the fact that yoghurt contains less lactose than milk. As a result, those who struggle to digest lactose generally find they tolerate yoghurt better than the milk from which it is derived.

Strained yoghurt is an even better option, as the straining process 'concentrates' the yoghurt (making it more substantial as a food) and also removes some of the sugar. Greek-style strained yoghurts are therefore preferred over regular yoghurt.

While yoghurt is a generally healthy food, 'fruit' yoghurts

should be avoided as they tend to contain heaps of added sugar and/or artificial sweeteners, and precious little fruit. Plain yoghurt is a healthier choice, though there's no reason why this cannot be made more tasty and interesting, not to mention nutritious, with foods such as berries, nuts and seeds.

Cream, like yoghurt, is generally well tolerated. Cheese is not particularly well tolerated by individuals who are dairy-sensitive, but sheep's and goat's forms of cheese (e.g. feta, haloumi, manchega, soft and hard goat's cheeses) are generally much better tolerated than cheese made from cow's milk. Cream and cheese are relatively protein- and fat-rich, low-carb foods, which makes them acceptable choices for those seeking to lose weight, despite their fattening reputation.

Ice cream is not recommended, at least in part on account of its high sugar content.

The nutritional attributes of butter were covered earlier. From a food-sensitivity perspective, butter is generally very well tolerated. This may have something to do with the fact that it is low in the protein and lactose elements that are usually at the root of food-sensitivity reactions.

Summary

- Plain yoghurt may be eaten freely.

- Sugar- or artificially sweetened yoghurts are to be avoided.

- Cream and cheese can be eaten in moderation, though goat's and sheep's cheese are preferred over cow's.

- Milk and ice cream should be avoided.

FOODS WITH ADDED SUGAR

Confectionery, sweet pastries, puddings, biscuits, cakes, doughnuts and the like should be avoided on account of their high-sugar nature. Many of these foods contain a lot of refined flour (generally high GI) as well as partially-hydrogenated fats. These foods should be avoided.

One sweet treat that might have some place in the diet is dark chocolate (70 per cent cocoa solids or more). Cocoa is actually quite a nutritious substance in its own right, and particularly rich in plant chemicals known as polyphenols that are linked with a reduced risk of heart disease. The darker the chocolate, the more cocoa it contains and, importantly, the less sugar. Also, compared to milk chocolate, people tend to eat less of it. More about this can be found in Chapter 6.

Summary

• **Foods with added sugar should be avoided.**

GRAINS

Generally speaking, grains such as wheat, oats, rye, barley, rice and corn have high GIs and GLs, and are not recommended. These foods, even in their wholegrain form, also offer little from a nutritional perspective. There is nothing that grains offer that cannot be found elsewhere in the diet, and in far healthier forms, too.

Summary

• **Grains should be avoided.**

OTHER FOODSTUFFS

Food containing artificial sweeteners (see Chapters 6 and 8), MSG (see Chapter 6) or partially-hydrogenated and trans fat (see Chapter 4) should be avoided. In the UK, there is no legal requirement for manufacturers to declare their products' trans fat content. However, the presence of partially-hydrogenated fat/oil/vegetable oil in a food is a sign that trans fats are likely to be present. The presence of a partially-hydrogenated fat in a food is, of course, a reason in itself not to consume that food.

Foods To Consume In Unlimited Quantity	Foods To Consume In Moderation	Foods To Avoid
Meat (unprocessed) and home-made burgers/patties/meatballs	Processed meats e.g. bacon, ham, salami, sausages	
Fish (especially oily fish such as salmon, mackerel, herring and sardines) and seafood	Tuna, marlin, swordfish	
Eggs		
Berries, avocado	Apples, pears, plums, citrus fruits (mango, pineapple and banana in more limited quantities)	dried fruit (except in small quantities)
Green vegetables, salad vegetables, onions	Squash, pumpkin, carrots, swede, parsnips, sweet potato	Potato
	Beans, lentils, peas and peanuts	
	Fermented soya products such as tempeh, natto and miso	Soya milk and soya products based on TVP and SPI

Foods To Consume In Unlimited Quantity	Foods To Consume In Moderation	Foods To Avoid
		Quorn
	Dark chocolate	Foods with added sugar such as soft drinks, confectionery, biscuits, cakes, pastries
Nuts and seeds		
Butter, olive oil, avocado oil, coconut oil	Sesame oil	Margarine
Plain yoghurt (especially strained)	Cream, cheese (goat's and sheep's cheeses preferred)	Sweetened yoghurt, milk, ice cream
		Foods with added sugar
		Grain-based foods such as bread, rice, pasta, breakfast cereals, crackers
		Foods containing MSG
		Foods containing artificial sweeteners
		Foods containing partially-hydrogenated fats

BACK TO BASICS

- In general, the diet should be made up of foods that are rich in protein and healthy fats, and low in carbohydrates that disrupt blood-sugar and insulin levels.

- Food additives, particularly MSG and artificial sweeteners, should be avoided.

- Foods rich in micronutrients, phytochemicals and soluble fibre should be emphasised in the diet.

- Meat is a highly nutritious food that is a good source of protein (which, amongst other things, can help sate the appetite), iron, zinc, B-vitamins, carnitine, leucine and monounsaturated fat.

- The evidence suggests that unprocessed meats are healthier than processed meats such as salami and bacon.

- Fish and seafood help provide the body with important nutrients like iodine and zinc. Some fish are a good source of the so-called omega-3 fats which have important benefits for the cardiovascular system and brain.

- Vegetarian diets are not inherently healthier than more omnivorous ones.

- Eggs are also a rich source of protein and nutrients such as monounsaturated fat, iron and B_{12}. Eating eggs does not have a strong link with heart disease.

- Fruit is a generally nutritious food, but is usually high in sugar, which can make it a problem if eaten in excess. Some of the best fruits include berries and avocado.

- Many vegetables that grow above ground such as lettuce, cabbage and broccoli are generally nutritious and of low-carbohydrate load.

- Some vegetables have higher carbohydrate content and should be eaten in moderation, including carrots, parsnips and squash.

- Potatoes generally have high glycaemic indices and tend to be lower in nutritional value than other vegetables, and should be avoided.

- Nuts and seeds are highly nutritious and seem to help protect against heart disease. Eating them does not appear to cause weight gain.

- Many vegetable oils are rich in omega-6 fats, which tend to be over-emphasised in the diet. Healthier sources of fat include olive oil, avocado oil and coconut oil.

- Butter is healthier than margarine.

- Beans and lentils may cause problems with food sensitivity and also contain compounds that have an 'anti-nutrient' effect. They should be eaten in moderation.

- Yoghurt is healthier than milk and cheese, and in its plain form can be eaten freely.

- Soya and Quorn have properties that do not make them ideal for human consumption.

- Foods with added sugar should be avoided.

- Grains, mainly on account of their tendency to disrupt blood-sugar and insulin levels, and their generally low nutritional status, should be avoided.

Chapter 8

LIQUID ASSETS

THE BEST BEVERAGES FOR WEIGHT AND WELLBEING

Effective fat loss and optimal health aren't just about what we eat, but also what we *drink*. So in this chapter we're going to be taking an in-depth look at the major beverages in the modern-day diet, and examine their appropriateness with regard to both weight and wellbeing. We will start with water – the most fundamental of fluids – before moving on to coffee, tea, fruit juice, soft drinks and alcohol. As with the preceding chapter, each fluid will be rated as something that may be drunk freely, in moderation, or not at all.

WATER – THE FORGOTTEN NUTRIENT

The adult human body is about two-thirds water, and this fact alone suggests that this fluid has an important part to play in health and wellbeing. Actually, all of our biochemical, physiological and neurological processes depend, to some degree, on water. For instance, water makes up the bulk of our blood volume. If we do not keep ourselves properly topped up with fluid, this may be reflected in a slightly reduced blood volume and blood pressure. The end result here is that our circulation will fail to deliver oxygen and nutrients to all our tissues and organs with optimal efficiency.

Circulation is key to ensuring proper detoxification of the body and elimination of waste through the kidneys. Even relatively mild dehydration might therefore increase the risk of toxic build-up in the body, which is likely to have a negative impact on our health and wellbeing. Water is also important for nerve-transmission in the body. Running low on fluid can therefore have consequences for brain function. Water basically helps all body and brain processes run that much more smoothly. No wonder, then, that while the human body can usually go a few weeks or even months without food, it can only manage a few days without water.

WHAT ARE THE BENEFITS OF DRINKING WATER?

Because water plays a critical role in the body's most fundamental processes, dehydration can manifest in a myriad of ways. Lethargy (of both body and mind) is a common symptom of dehydration. Individuals generally find that getting a bit more water into their system buoys up their mental and physical energy, often within half an hour or so.

Another quite common consequence of dehydration is headache. One theory about how this happens is that running low on fluid can cause the membranes that cover the brain (called meninges) to exert some downward pressure, which is sensed as pain. Whether this is true or not I can't say definitively, but one thing I know for sure is that many individuals with 'mystery' headaches end up banishing them simply by drinking more water.

Dehydration can cause constipation, too. When the body runs dry, it does its utmost to extract every last drop of water from waste matter in the large colon. The end result can be a bit like cork stuck in the neck of a wine bottle. Keeping well hydrated is often a crucial tactic in keeping our bowels moving along nicely.

On top of this, there is evidence linking higher water consumption with a reduced risk of heart disease[1] and some forms of cancer.[2,3]

For optimal health and well-being, it pays to keep topped up with water.

CAN DRINKING WATER HELP FAT LOSS?

'Detox' regimes are often recommended as a path to weight loss, and a major component of such regimes is water. While the idea that simply downing more water might assist in the search for a slimmer body may seem unlikely, there does actually seem to be some scientific support for this practice.

For example, it has been found that cells that are dehydrated do not take up glucose very efficiently[4]– something that could cause the metabolism to stall. Also, studies show that when the blood is made more dilute, fatty breakdown in the body (lipolysis) is enhanced.[5,6]

This evidence suggests that there is some support for the notion that keeping well hydrated can assist in our quest to shed fat.

HOW MUCH WATER DO WE NEED?

Our need for water is dependent on many different factors including propensity to sweating, size, activity levels, temperature, humidity and how much water might be taken in from, say, fruits and vegetables. What this means is that it's very difficult to make blanket recommendations about water intake. Because of this, it's better for us to tune into personal indicators of our state of hydration.

Thirst is not a good indicator, as by the time the body is thirsty it is often quite dehydrated indeed. A good gauge, though, to the state of our hydration is the colour of our urine.[7] Essentially, the paler our urine is, the better our state of hydration. *The aim is to drink enough water to keep your urine pale yellow in colour throughout the day.* If your urine colour strays into darker tones, particularly if this is accompanied by a noticeable smell, then it's time to step up your water intake. Most individuals, most of the time, need to drink in the order of 2–3 litres of water each day to maintain a good state of hydration and pale urine.

KEEP WATER BY YOU

For many people, the idea of drinking 2 or 3 litres of water a day seems like quite a feat. The one big piece of advice I have about getting plenty of water into the body each day is: *keep water by you.* When individuals have water in front of them, they tend to drink a lot more than if they repeatedly need to get it from, say, the fridge or the water cooler down the end of the corridor.

If you're doing the gardening, keep a bottle of water with you. Put a bottle of water on your desk at work, and make sure there is water available in meetings. Put a bottle of water in the car and carry one in your briefcase, rucksack or sports bag when you are out and about. If you keep water by you, you're likely to get through decent quantities of the stuff (but if you don't, you probably *won't*).

Summary

• **Water may be drunk freely.**

HERBAL AND FRUIT TEAS, TEA AND COFFEE

Herbal and fruit teas are an alternative to water for those seeking to maintain good levels of hydration throughout the day. In addition, some of these beverages may have some therapeutic benefit for the body. Fennel and peppermint, for instance, may aid digestion, while chamomile can aid restful sleep.

Tea

Tea comes in two main forms – black (regular tea) and green. Basically, black tea is made from allowing green tea to undergo oxidation. Both main forms of tea contain caffeine and other stimulants, as well as disease-protective compounds known as polyphenols, which have 'antioxidant' activity. This means they have the capacity to neutralise the effects of damaging, disease-causing molecules called 'free radicals'. In general terms, green tea contains less caffeine and has more antioxidant capacity than black tea.

Black Tea and Health

There is quite a lot of research which links black tea consumption with a reduced risk of heart disease. A review in the *European Journal of Clinical Nutrition* found that three or more cups of black tea seem to be what is required to get this benefit.[8] The review also found that, despite the fact that tea contains some caffeine and other substances which have a diuretic effect (meaning they stimulate urine production), drinking tea did not generally cause dehydration in the body. Tea drinking has also been associated with a reduced risk of stroke in men.[9]

Green Tea and Health

Green tea has also been associated with a reduced risk of heart disease.[10] This benefit is thought to be, at least in part, due to one of the polyphenols found in green tea going by the name of epigallocatechin-3-gallate (EGCG). This compound has also been found to have a number of cancer-protective actions in the body, including an ability to help in the deactivation of cancer-causing chemicals (carcinogens). There is evidence to suggest that regular consumption of green tea is associated with a reduced risk of some forms of cancer.[11]

CAN GREEN TEA HELP FAT-BURNING IN THE BODY?

Some research has explored the role that green tea may play in the metabolism of fat in the body. In one study, giving men green tea extract (containing 350 mg of a compound found in green tea known as epigallocatechin-3-gallate – or EGCG)[12] was found to enhance fat metabolism by 17 per cent.

In another study,[13] overweight men were treated with 300 mg of EGCG or placebo for just two days. EGCG ingestion was found to stimulate the metabolism of fat after a meal.

In another study, overweight men were asked to drink catechin-rich tea (EGCG is part of a group of compounds referred to as 'catechins') or low-catechin tea for 12 weeks.[14] The catechin-rich tea led to significant reductions in body weight, waist size and fat mass. The total catechin amount supplied by the 'active' tea was 690 mg a day – which equates to about 5–6 cups of green tea.[15]

In a similar study,[16] individuals were given a daily beverage containing 625 mg of catechins for a period of 12 weeks. Another group, who acted as 'controls', were given a drink without catechins. Over the 12-week study period, individuals were advised to partake in three hours or more of moderate-intensity activity each week. At the beginning and end of the study, participants underwent a variety of measurements including body composition and the 'abdominal fat area' (a measure of the amount of fat in and around the abdomen).

The results of this study found that changes in overall fat levels (fat mass) in the body were not different between the two groups. However, fat area in the abdomen was significantly lower in the group consuming the catechin-laced beverage. As an added bonus, levels of blood fats known as triglycerides were significantly lower in the catechin-consuming group, too.

A word of caution: a recently published study found evidence that green tea components appear to block the action of the chemotherapy drug bortezomib (Velcade).[17] Those taking this drug should consult their doctors regarding green tea use.

Coffee and Health

Coffee has a reputation as the devil's brew, but the evidence suggests this demonised beverage may well have a range of positive benefits for health. It is true that coffee is naturally rich in caffeine, which in excess has the capacity to induce issues such as mood change and insomnia. On the other hand, coffee is very rich in disease-protective 'antioxidant' substances including polyphenols.

Drinking coffee is actually very consistently associated with a reduced risk of diabetes[18-20] and metabolic syndrome.[21] Its consumption is also associated with a reduced risk of stroke in men.[22]

Coffee and Dementia

Some evidence also links coffee drinking with a reduced risk of dementia including Alzheimer's disease.[23,24] In this study, individuals drinking 3–5 cups of coffee a day were found to have only roughly a third of the risk of developing dementia compared to individuals drinking little or no coffee.

It is possible that the antioxidants in coffee help protect brain cells from the damage wreaked by chemical entities known as 'free radicals'. Also, we know that coffee consumption is associated with a reduced risk of diabetes, and diabetes is a risk factor for dementia (essentially because it increases the risk of 'vascular dementia', which causes impaired blood supply to the brain). It is also possible that coffee may provide some protection against dementia through its ability to deliver caffeine to the body: an animal study has found that giving caffeine to mice with Alzheimer's disease improved their brain function.[25] Caffeine also reduces the production of the protein beta-amyloid – deposits of which are typically found in the brains of Alzheimer's disease sufferers.

THE PRIMAL PRINCIPLE – COFFEE AND TEA

The idea that tea and coffee might be beneficial to health may not seem to make sense from an evolutionary perspective. After all, these beverages are relatively recent additions to the human diet. However, the main constituent of these drinks is water. Of course, that won't always guarantee that a beverage is healthy. For example, the prime constituent of a solution of arsenic and cyanide is also water, but it still wouldn't be good to drink. But let's not forget that coffee comes from a bean and tea from a leaf – both of which are naturally-occurring. Not all things in nature are good to consume (e.g. poisonous mushrooms), but when tea and coffee are analysed chemically, they both turn out to be very rich in health-promoting polyphenols. When such substances are infused into some hot water, it's perhaps not that surprising that the resulting beverages turn out to have benefits for health.

Summary

- Herb and fruit teas may be drunk freely.
- Caffeinated tea and coffee may be drunk in moderation.
- Naturally decaffeinated tea and coffee may be drunk freely.

WHAT DOES 'MODERATION' MEAN?

The same 'moderation' rules apply to drinks as to food: wherever possible, opt for drinks such as water, herb and fruit teas, and naturally decaffeinated tea or coffee. However, from time to time you can deviate from this and have, say, a cup of caffeinated coffee. In the initial stages of changing your diet, avoid doing this more than once a day. In the long term you can relax this, but aim to ensure that at least 80 per cent of your fluid intake comes from beverages from the 'consume in unlimited quantity' list (see page **150**).

SUGARY SOFT DRINKS

Sugary soft drinks generally contain sugar in the form of sucrose (table sugar) or something known as high-fructose corn syrup. Each molecule of sucrose (which comes mainly from sugar cane and sugar beet) is made of a molecule each of glucose and fructose. High-fructose corn syrup also contains glucose and fructose, in roughly equal measure. Both sucrose and high-fructose corn syrup have the capacity to disrupt blood-sugar levels in a way that can stimulate the manufacture of fat and at the same time stall the body's fat-burning abilities (see Chapter 3 for more on the biochemical mechanisms involved here).

In theory, then, sugary soft drinks might possibly be helping to fuel the rise in rates of obesity seen in countries eating a typical Western diet. In the USA, assessment of the nation's diet (via National Health and Nutrition Examination Surveys) have revealed that the explosion of obesity that started in the 1970s and continues to this day has been mirrored by an increase in carbohydrate intake, principally from added sugar. It is perhaps interesting to note that, at the same time, the proportion of the diet contributed by fat has *fallen*.

There has been particular concern that *drinking* sugar, in the form of sugary soft drinks, say, is more hazardous to weight than eating it. Sugary soft drinks allow the potential to get a lot of sugar-laden calories into the body very quickly. It also seems that when sugar is drunk, the body is less likely to compensate with a reduced intake of other foodstuffs than if that sugar were eaten.

In 2006, US researchers assessed 30 relevant studies in the area, and concluded that '... greater consumption of SSBs [sugar-sweetened beverages] is associated with weight gain and obesity.'[26] There is also evidence that added sugar in the diet can contribute to cardiovascular disease (e.g. heart attacks and strokes).[27] In addition, sugar can have other adverse effects on health including suppression of the immune system,[28-30] nutrient depletion[31-34] and the induction of insulin resistance (a precursor of type 2 diabetes).[35]

It's important to bear in mind, I think, just how much sugar there is in soft drinks. Many contain the equivalent of 9 teaspoons of sugar in a 330-ml can. A half-litre bottle offers about 14 teaspoons of sugar. In addition, some soft drinks include caffeine (which stimulates urine production) and salt. The caffeine and salt in some soft drinks can trigger thirst, and therefore a desire for more of the same. Clearly, those looking to do what they can to optimise their health and weight should avoid sugary soft drinks.

IS FRUCTOSE A HEALTHY ALTERNATIVE TO REGULAR SUGAR?

Fructose is often touted as a healthy alternative to sucrose (table sugar). This is based on the fact that it's found in fruit (which itself has an eminently healthy image) and does not raise blood glucose levels immediately after it is eaten. However, the reality is that there is evidence that we need to be wary of this 'healthy' form of sugar. In one relevant study, men were fed a fructose-rich diet for four weeks.[36] This led to a very significant increase in the levels of blood fats known as 'triglycerides' (higher levels of which are associated with metabolic syndrome and heightened heart disease risk). Also, the fructose-rich diet was found to cause an increase in blood-glucose levels (contrary to traditional wisdom).

Other evidence shows that fructose can impair the body's ability to handle sugar, as well as reduce the effectiveness of insulin.[37] A review of the relationship between sugar and cardiovascular disease[38] cites evidence which links the consumption of fructose with various ills including type 2 diabetes, raised blood pressure and obesity.

In one study, feeding individuals fructose-rich drinks was found to bring about detrimental effects in terms of insulin sensitivity, blood-fat levels, fasting sugar levels and fatty accumulation.[39] There is good evidence that fructose, as added to food, has the capacity to be detrimental to health and weight, and should be avoided.

Summary

- **Sugary soft drinks should be avoided.**

ARTIFICIALLY SWEETENED BEVERAGES

Artificial sweeteners are sweet but contain virtually no calories, and therefore are often promoted as a 'healthy' alternative to sugar, particularly for those looking to lose weight. But you may recall that in an earlier chapter (Satisfaction Guaranteed) we learned that artificial sweeteners have the capacity to stimulate the appetite, and appear to cause obesity in animals.

To know for sure whether artificial sweeteners are better than sugar for weight control they would need to be subjected to 'randomised controlled trials'. This essentially means taking a group of individuals and randomly assigning them to a diet containing either artificial sweeteners or sugar. In an ideal world, neither the participants nor the scientists conducting the study would know who was consuming what. At the end of a predetermined period, the 'code' would be 'cracked' and an assessment made of who did better in the weight stakes (if anyone).

This sort of study is used for pharmaceutical agents to prove their effectiveness (or otherwise) and validate them as fit for purpose. However, despite all the talk about how artificial sweeteners are the 'healthy' choice for weight, there has not been a single randomised controlled trial in the scientific literature attesting to the weight-loss 'benefits' of these sweeteners.

The other thing to bear in mind is that artificial sweeteners are, by definition, alien to nature. Theoretically, at least, we might expect them to have adverse effects on health. And science bears this out. For example, saccharin has been found to induce cancer in animals. So does aspartame. In one study, Italian researchers fed aspartame in a variety of doses to rats over the long term.[40] Rats consuming aspartame were found to be at significantly increased risk of several forms of cancer including lymphoma and leukaemia (cancer of the white blood cells). An increased risk of these conditions was found even at levels of aspartame intake lower than the official upper limit for humans. While in Europe intakes of 40 mg of aspartame per kg of body weight per day are considered safe, an increased risk in cancer was seen in rats consuming just half this amount. Aspartame has also been linked with a range of adverse effects on health including headaches[41,42] and depression.[43]

The manufacturers of aspartame, and the trade organisations and scientists that represent them, will, of course, point to plenty of studies that apparently attest to aspartame's safety. There are, however, also plenty that suggest it poses genuine hazards for health. A review of relevant studies[44] shows that while 100 per cent of industry-funded studies conclude that aspartame is safe, 92 per cent of independently funded research identifies aspartame as a potential cause of harmful effects. On health grounds, I advise avoiding artificial sweeteners.

Summary

• Artificially sweetened drinks should be avoided.

FRUIT JUICE

Fruit juices are often seen as healthy drinks that are roughly equivalent, nutritionally speaking, to whole fruit. However, in juicing a fruit, many nutritious elements – in particular fibre and also a proportion of nutrients – are left behind. The sugar concentration of fruit juices (even unsweetened ones) is essentially the same (or even higher) than that of sugary soft drinks. Much of this sugar can come in the form of fructose, which has traditionally enjoyed a healthy reputation. However, as we have learned (see page **143**), fructose has the capacity to induce weight gain as well as having other adverse effects on health.

In one study, an increase in fruit juice consumption of one serving a day was associated with an 18 per cent increased risk of diabetes.[45] Fruit juices are not a good choice for individuals seeking to optimise their weight and health.

Another option for fruit-based drinks is the 'smoothie'. These drinks are generally better than juices, as many of them contain whole fruit mashed up. I think smoothies are mostly a healthier option than fruit juices, but they are still intensely sugary and need to be consumed with care. I advise that they are drunk in moderation, and not at all until you are near to achieving your weight and health goals.

Summary

• Fruit juice should be avoided.
• Smoothies may be consumed in moderation.

ALCOHOL

Alcoholic beverages are generally a source of carbohydrate which, remember, is a prime driver of weight gain. Perhaps unsurprisingly, several studies show that higher alcohol intakes are associated with greater body weight. Many studies have also found an association between higher alcohol intakes and increased risk of abdominal obesity.[46-48]

For a given amount of alcohol, beer and cider contain much more carb than wine (they're not called 'beer bellies' for nothing). Of the wines, red wine contains, generally speaking, less carbohydrate than white. So, if your goal is to lose fat effectively, drink as little as possible, and when you do drink, perhaps limit yourself to a glass of red wine with your evening meal.

Is Moderate Drinking Healthy?

Moderate drinking is often promoted as something that is 'healthy', mainly on account of the fact that this habit is associated with a reduced risk of heart disease. However, in relevant studies, individuals in the teetotal group may include, for instance, reformed alcoholics. As alcoholism is likely to lead to long-term damage to the heart, this might artificially push up the heart disease rates seen in teetotal groups. Also, one reason why people may be abstaining from drink is that they have been diagnosed with heart disease and therefore have been advised to cut out alcohol or have decided for themselves to take this step. Basically, this can bias the results of the studies and make it seem that abstaining from alcohol is not as healthy as it might be in reality.

Another major flaw of the oft-quoted alcohol research is that it has often focused only on heart disease. This is an important health condition, but it accounts for only about a quarter of deaths. What about the other three-quarters?

As it happens, alcohol is known to increase the risk of other conditions that can prove fatal, including liver disease and cancer. Therefore, to make a decent judgement on the effects of alcohol on health we shouldn't really be focusing only on heart disease, but on the overall risk of death.

When researchers have focused on overall mortality, a slightly different picture from the 'healthy tipple' image of alcohol emerges. One study found that in men up to the age of 34, the optimal amount of alcohol to drink was none at all.[49] In this study there seemed to be some benefits of alcohol consumption later in life – the optimal intake being a shade over 1 unit a day. As a sometime drinker myself, I take no satisfaction in imparting this news, but it seems that the 'benefits' of drinking alcohol have been somewhat overstated.

EASY WAYS TO DRINK LESS

While I think the 'benefits' of alcohol have been overplayed, I am also of the belief that not everything that passes our lips need be explicitly healthy. There are other reasons (for example, taste and conviviality) for consuming foodstuffs, and this includes alcohol. However, the fact remains that any more than very moderate drinking is likely to jeopardise your weight-loss efforts, so it can help to take steps to moderate your drinking in the long term.

One tactic that works well here is to match each alcoholic drink (e.g. glass of wine) with a glass of water. This usually leads to less wine being drunk, and also 'dilutes' any negative effects the alcohol may have. Plus, more water is going into the body, which is broadly healthy.

Two other strategies for containing alcohol consumption are to avoid getting too hungry or thirsty. Avoiding thirst is an obvious tactic, but it is less well recognised that hunger can be a major driver of alcohol intake, particularly early in the evening. Many people look to alcohol to get themselves out of the low-sugar hole dug by eating a sandwich for lunch and then nothing more before dinner.

Matching each alcoholic drink with one of water, and avoiding undue hunger and thirst, are all effective tactics for reducing alcohol intake without feeling deprived.

Is Red Wine Any Better?

Red wine, more than any other form of alcohol, has often been recommended as 'healthy'. Much scientific focus has been put on a constituent of red grapes known as resveratrol, the actions of which in the body would help to explain red wine's proposed benefits for the heart. However, a close look at the evidence reveals that wine drinkers, compared to those who generally choose other forms of alcohol such as beer and spirits, tend to eat healthier diets and smoke less, too.[50-52] These studies actually show it's not the red wine *per se*, but these other factors associated with drinking red wine that account for the apparent 'benefits'.

Summary

• **Alcohol should be drunk in moderation. Red wine, on account of its generally low-carbohydrate content, is to be preferred over white wine and beer.**

Beverages To Consume In Unlimited Quantity	Beverages To Consume In Moderation	Beverages To Avoid
Water		
Herb and fruit teas		
Naturally decaffeinated coffee and tea	Caffeinated coffee and tea	
	Smoothies	Fruit juice
		Sugary and artificially sweetened soft drinks
	Red wine	White wine, beer, cider

BACK TO BASICS

- Water plays an important role in physiological and neurological processes in the body and brain.

- Maintaining hydration can enhance energy and prevent symptoms such as headache and constipation.

- There is evidence that drinking more water may enhance fat loss.

- Enough water should be drunk to ensure the urine is pale yellow in colour throughout the course of the day.

- Herb and fruit teas make a healthy alternative to water.

- Tea consumption is linked with a reduced risk of cardiovascular disease, and green tea consumption with a reduced risk of cancer.

- Green tea extracts have been found to stimulate fat metabolism and fat loss.

- Coffee consumption is linked with a reduced risk of metabolic syndrome, diabetes and dementia.

- Soft drinks loaded with sugar are likely to have adverse effects on health and weight.

- Fructose is not a healthy alternative to regular sugar (sucrose).

- Artificial sweeteners are not a healthy alternative to sugar, and neither is there any good evidence that they assist weight loss.

- Fruit juice is intensely sugary and is not recommended for those seeking to optimise their health and weight.

- The benefits of alcohol have been generally overstated.

- Alcohol is associated with higher body weight and abdominal obesity.

- Balancing alcohol intake with water is very likely to reduce the negative impact alcohol can have on health.

Chapter 9

MAKE A MEAL OF IT

RECIPES, MEAL PLANS AND PRACTICAL TIPS FOR HEALTHY EATING SUCCESS

So far this book has mainly focused on the theory regarding what to eat, and what not to eat, for fat-loss success. This chapter is about how to put that theory into practice.

Here you will find a range of meal and snack ideas that are consistent with the nutritional principles you've learned. Recipes are included, too, many of which do not require much in the way of cooking skills (including many that can be prepared in about 15 minutes or less). Vegetarian (V) and fish (F) recipes have been marked as such.

At the end of the chapter you can find practical information and advice on how to approach each of the three main meals of the day, as well as snacking. Here I've included information about the best options, both in and out of the home, including practical options that you can take from home to eat elsewhere should you wish. Suggestions about how to handle eating out effectively are also given.

BREAKFASTS
Yoghurt, Berries and Nuts (V)
Breadless Scotch Egg
Scrambled Eggs, Indian Style (V)
Fried Breakfast
Chorizo, Goat's Cheese and Red Pepper Omelette
Scrambled Eggs and Smoked Salmon (F)
Poached Eggs with Spinach (V)

MEALS
Tuna and Egg Salad (F)
Home-made Beefburger with Tomato and Rocket Salad
Tomato Soup and Parmesan Cheese (V)
Sausages and Cabbage
Griddled Lamb or Steak with Tomato, Red Onion and Coriander Salad
Prawn/Crayfish and Mango Salad (F)
Roast Chicken with Piri Piri Sauce
Prawn/Beef/Pork/Chicken Stir-fry (F-prawn)
Bolognese with Cabbage 'Pasta'
Spicy Seafood Stew (F)
Chorizo, Chestnut, Manchego and Coriander Salad
Classic Chilli
Salmon Niçoise Salad (F)
Venison Casserole
Frittata (V option)
Roast Vegetable and Goat's Cheese Stack (V)
Bean Nut Roast with Pease Pudding (V)
Monkfish with Ginger and Lime (F)
Mackerel with Garlic and Rosemary Cooked in Foil (F)

BREAKFASTS

YOGHURT, BERRIES AND NUTS (V)
🕐15 minutes or less

plain, full-fat yoghurt (preferably strained)
handful of berries (fresh or frozen and defrosted)
chopped or ground nuts (e.g. almonds, pecans, walnuts, hazelnuts)

Take the yoghurt, berries and nuts of your choice. The quantities you use here are really down to the level of your hunger and taste. As a rough guide, about 4 dessertspoons of yoghurt, 2 dessertspoons of nuts and 2 dessertspoons of berries will make a satisfying breakfast. This mix of foods can also make a good snack or even dessert, in which case smaller quantities will usually suffice.

BREADLESS SCOTCH EGG
6-8 eggs (hardboiled)
500 g pork mince
salt
pepper
light olive oil

Take each hard-boiled egg and wrap in seasoned pork mince (aim to get the mince 1-1.5 cm in thickness). Leave to chill in the fridge for at least 2 hours – if you skip this step, the scotch eggs will tend to disintegrate when they are cooked. Deep fry in oil until golden brown. Remove from oil and allow to drain and cool on some kitchen roll.

If you like these, I recommend making them in batches of 6 or 8 (they keep well in the fridge in an airtight container or wrapped in foil). One or two will really set you up for the day, or also make a handy and tasty snack.

Variations

Think about adding some herbs and spices to the pork mince. Finely chopped garlic and chilli work well if you like these flavours. Another alternative is to add some finely chopped bacon and/or small cubes of black pudding.

If you don't eat pork, you might like to use another meat such as lamb or beef.

SCRAMBLED EGGS, INDIAN STYLE (V)

⏲ 15 minutes or less
Serves 1

olive oil
1 medium red onion, finely chopped
½–1 bird's-eye chilli pepper, deseeded and finely chopped
1 medium tomato, chopped
3 medium eggs, beaten
salt and pepper
handful of fresh coriander, roughly chopped

Heat the oil in a frying pan and add the onion and chilli pepper; cook until the onion is softened. Add the chopped tomato and continue cooking for a few minutes. Turn the heat down and add the eggs, keeping them moving with a wooden spoon or spatula. Add salt and pepper to taste, and cook eggs to the consistency of your choice. Near the end of the cooking, add the fresh coriander.

Serve alone or with grilled or fried tomatoes and/or mushrooms.

FRIED BREAKFAST

Take your pick from eggs, bacon, sausage, black pudding, tomatoes and mushrooms, with a small dollop of ketchup, brown sauce or mustard. Just avoid the bread.

CHORIZO, GOAT'S CHEESE AND RED PEPPER OMELETTE

⏱ 15 minutes or less
Serves 1

olive oil
½ red onion, finely chopped
¼ red pepper, diced
½ bird's-eye chilli, deseeded and finely chopped (optional)
chorizo, diced or cut into small squares
2 eggs, beaten
50 g soft goat's cheese

Heat the oil in a small frying pan and add the onion, red pepper and chilli (if desired) and cook until the onion is soft. Add the chorizo and cook for a further minute. Add this mix to the beaten eggs, and crumble most of the goat's cheese into the mix. Add more oil to the frying pan, heat and add the mix back to the pan. Crumble the remainder of the goat's cheese on top. Once the underside is cooked (this should take a few minutes), finish the top off under the grill.

Variation

Fresh coriander, added either into the omelette and/or sprinkled on top after cooking, works well with this mix of flavours.

SCRAMBLED EGGS WITH SMOKED SALMON (F)

🕐 15 minutes or less
Serves 1

butter
3 eggs, beaten
salt
pepper
50 g smoked salmon (cut into thin strips)

Heat the butter in a small saucepan until melted. Keep the heat low. Add the eggs and keep them moving. Add salt and pepper to taste, and cook the eggs to the desired consistency. Throw in the smoked salmon near the end of the cooking process.

Serve with grilled/fried mushrooms and/or tomatoes.

POACHED EGGS WITH SPINACH (V)

Serves 1

2 eggs
white wine vinegar
butter
1 clove garlic, finely chopped
200 g spinach
1 tsp lemon juice
salt
pepper

Poach the eggs in boiling water that has had some vinegar added, for about 3 minutes. Turn the heat off, put a lid on the saucepan, and leave for 3-4 minutes.

Meanwhile, cook the spinach: melt some butter in a saucepan, add the garlic and the spinach and pour in the lemon juice. Stir and cook for about 1 minute. Season with salt and pepper. Cook for 1 minute more. Put the spinach on a plate and add the poached eggs on top.

Variation

You might want to jazz up this dish with some Hollandaise sauce. Here's how to make it:

100 g butter
3 large egg yolks
salt
1 tbsps lemon juice
dash of Tabasco sauce or something similar (optional)
2 tbsps hot water

Heat the butter in a saucepan until foamy. Do not allow it to brown (if you do, the butter's overcooked and you'll need to start again). While the butter is melting, beat the egg yolks and add salt and lemon juice, and hot pepper sauce (if desired).

Turn the butter to a low heat and gradually add the egg mixture to this, whisking all the time. Once all the eggs are in, add hot water, a little at a time, to achieve the consistency of single cream. Serve immediately on top of the poached eggs.

MEALS

TUNA AND EGG SALAD (F)
⏱ 15 minutes or less
Serves 2–4

1 red pepper
2 cans of tuna, drained
1 can kidney or flageolet beans (drained and rinsed)
1 medium red onion, finely chopped
2 cloves garlic, finely chopped
3 medium tomatoes, chopped
1 handful fresh coriander, roughly chopped
olive oil
lemon juice
salt
black pepper
2 eggs, hard-boiled

Place the red pepper under a hot grill until blackened. Turn the pepper and keep grilling until it is almost completely black. You can also do this by placing the red pepper on a lit gas ring and turning it periodically. Plunge into cold water and remove skin. Cut the pepper into thin slices.

Mix the pepper slices with the tuna, kidney beans, onion, garlic, tomatoes and coriander. Dress with olive oil and lemon juice, and season with salt and pepper. Transfer to a serving dish. Slice the hardboiled eggs into quarters, lengthways. Arrange the egg quarters around the edge of the salad and serve.

Variations
This dish can be made with other types of fish, such as canned mackerel or salmon.

HOME-MADE BEEFBURGER WITH TOMATO AND ROCKET SALAD
🕐 15 minutes or less
Serves 3–4

500 g beef mince
100 g Parmesan cheese, finely grated
2 cloves garlic, finely chopped
salt
pepper
olive oil
tomato, sliced
rocket leaves
Parmesan shavings

Mix the beef mince with the Parmesan cheese and garlic. Season with salt and pepper. Shape this mix into large-ish patties. Shallow fry in olive oil. While the patties are cooking, assemble the salad: start with a layer of tomato on a plate, add a mound of rocket leaves on top of this. Cover with Parmesan shavings and then drizzle with olive oil. Season with salt and pepper to taste. Once the burgers are done, put on top of the salad.

TOMATO SOUP AND PARMESAN CHEESE (V)
🕐 15 minutes or less

fresh tomato soup, preferably with no added sugar (can be sourced in a supermarket or deli)
fresh Parmesan cheese, grated

Take a fresh tomato-based soup, preferably with no added sugar. Add a good amount of grated fresh Parmesan cheese.

Accompany with salad dressed in olive oil and vinegar or lemon juice.

SAUSAGES AND CABBAGE
🕐 15 minutes or less

olive oil
good-quality sausages
cabbage (e.g. Savoy cabbage)
butter
salt
pepper
mustard

Grill or shallow fry the sausages. Steam or boil some shredded cabbage. Butter the cabbage and season with salt and pepper as required. Add sausages and serve with English, French or wholegrain mustard.

MISS MASH?

A sausage-based meal can, for some, seem somehow incomplete without mashed potato. The problem is, mashed potato tends to cause considerable blood-sugar and insulin disruption, and is therefore far from ideal for those seeking to shed fat. An alternative, though, is mashed cauliflower. Steam or boil the cauliflower until well done and then mash with butter, salt and pepper. This can make a great accompaniment to sausages as well as other foods including fish and chops. It can also be used as an alternative topping for shepherd's pie.

GRIDDLED LAMB OR STEAK WITH TOMATO, RED ONION AND CORIANDER SALAD

🕐 15 minutes or less

lamb steak, lamb chops or steak
salt
pepper
tomatoes, roughly chopped
red onion, finely chopped
fresh coriander, roughly chopped
olive oil
balsamic vinegar

Get a griddle pan very hot and sear the lamb or steak. Season with salt and pepper. While cooking, in a bowl mix the tomatoes, onion and coriander together in amounts and proportions to suit your taste. Dress with olive oil and a dash of balsamic vinegar. When the meat is done to your liking, serve alongside the salad.

Variation

The salad here goes well with fish, say trout or salmon. Fish is best not put on a griddle (if it sticks it will tend to disintegrate). Use a grill, or fry in some olive oil or butter.

PRAWN/CRAYFISH AND MANGO SALAD (F)
🕐 15 minutes or less

green salad leaves
prawns (peeled) and/or crayfish pieces or seafood sticks
ripe mango, cut into pieces
olive oil
garlic, finely chopped
lemon juice
salt
pepper

Put the salad leaves in a salad/serving bowl. Add the prawns/crayfish/seafood sticks and ripe mango. Make a dressing using the oil, garlic and a squeeze of lemon juice. Add salt and pepper to taste. Mix up the dressing with a fork, spoon or small whisk and then pour over the salad.

ROAST CHICKEN WITH PIRI PIRI SAUCE
Serves 4

olive oil
white wine (red wine will do, if it's all you have)
hot Piri Piri sauce (available in most supermarkets)
3 medium onions, peeled and sliced
1 small chicken
lemon (optional)
salt
black pepper

Mix the olive oil and white wine (half and half). You need the total volume to come to about 2 mugfulls. To this, add a few shakes of the hot Piri Piri sauce (the hotter and spicier you like your food, the more you should add). Whisk these ingredients together.

Place the onions in the bottom of a roasting dish and put the chicken (remove the giblets first) on top. Pour the olive oil, wine and Piri Piri mixture over the bird and put some inside the bird as well. If you want, you can add a lemon (cut into two pieces) inside the bird. Season the chicken with salt and freshly ground black pepper.

Roast in a hot oven according to instructions (usually 20 minutes per 500 kg plus a further 20 minutes). When done, leave to rest for 10 minutes under aluminium foil, and serve with buttered cabbage and/or other green vegetables.

PRAWN/BEEF/PORK/CHICKEN STIR-FRY (F-PRAWN)

⊕ 15 minutes or less
(use quantities to suit taste and volume required)

sesame oil
prawns (raw or cooked), thinly sliced beef or pork, or chicken cut into cubes or strips
ginger, thinly sliced
garlic, thinly sliced
sesame oil
bird's-eye chilli, finely chopped
bean sprouts, spring onions and carrots (thinly sliced), onions, peppers (alternatively, use one or two bags of pre-prepared 'stir-fry' vegetables)
soy sauce (optional)

Heat some sesame oil in a wok or deep frying pan, add the prawns (if raw) or meat and cook. Prawns cook very quickly. The meat needs to be cooked through. Remove the prawns/meat from the pan and put to one side. Heat some more oil and add the remaining ingredients. Cook until done to your liking (generally 3–7 minutes). Add the prawns/meat near the end, to heat through, and then serve.

Please note that stir-fries are traditionally seasoned with soy sauce. This is a source of MSG. See Chapter 6 for more about why this food ingredient is best avoided. This is particularly the case if you feel you may be sensitive to MSG (symptoms can include headaches, palpitations, nerve pain and insomnia). If you can enjoy your stir-fry without it, then my advice is to leave soy sauce out of the recipe. However, if you feel you need soy sauce for taste purposes, then make do with as little as possible.

BOLOGNESE WITH CABBAGE 'PASTA'
Serves 2–4

olive oil
2 large onions, peeled and chopped
2–3 cloves garlic, finely chopped
500 g beef mince
1–2 cans chopped tomatoes
tomato purée
red wine (a good slug)
fresh or dried oregano
salt
pepper
1 large cabbage, cut into ribbons
butter
Parmesan cheese, grated (optional)

Heat the olive oil in a sturdy, thick-bottomed pan. Add the onions and garlic and cook until softened. Add the mince and cook thoroughly, chopping it up with a wooden spoon or spatula. Add the canned tomatoes, some tomato purée, red wine and oregano. Mix thoroughly and leave to simmer.

This will be ready in about half an hour – stir occasionally. Add salt and pepper to taste.

Near the end of the cooking, steam the shredded cabbage. Ensure the cabbage is not overcooked or soft. Dress the cabbage with some butter or olive oil. Put the cabbage on a plate or in a bowl (this is the 'pasta') and add the 'Bolognese'/meat sauce on top. Add some freshly grated Parmesan cheese, if desired.

SPICY SEAFOOD STEW (F)
Serves 4–6

1 kg mixed seafood (frozen)
1 large onion, chopped
3 cloves garlic, finely chopped
1–2 bird's-eye chilli peppers, finely chopped
olive oil
1–2 cans chopped tomatoes
white wine (a good slug)
100 g chorizo, chopped
fresh coriander, roughly chopped
salt
pepper
lemon juice

Rinse the seafood in cold water. Cook the onion, garlic and chilli in the olive oil in a sturdy, large pan until softened and light brown. Add the chopped tomatoes and wine to this, and heat through. Now add the seafood and chorizo and cook over a medium heat for about 15 minutes. Season with salt and pepper and add lemon juice to taste. Add the coriander at the end of the cooking and mix through. Leave some coriander to use as garnish. Serve with a mixed, dressed salad.

CHORIZO, CHESTNUT, MANCHEGO AND CORIANDER SALAD

🕐 15 minutes or less

Serves 2

This salad has obvious Spanish influences and is delicious in all seasons. It takes just 5 minutes to put together.

8 whole chestnuts (fresh chestnuts in season, but otherwise organic, vacuum-packed chestnuts are fine)
12 thick (about 3-mm) slices of chorizo
rocket leaves (a good handful)
fresh coriander leaves (a good handful)
Manchego cheese (shavings)
olive oil
juice of half a lemon

Heat a dry pan and add the chestnuts. Cook until golden brown, and then place on a plate. In the same pan and on a medium heat, add the sliced chorizo and cook until golden brown. Build a salad of rocket leaves and sprigs of coriander. Add the chestnuts and the chorizo, and place on a serving dish. Top the salad with shavings of Manchego cheese and drizzle with olive oil and lemon juice.

CLASSIC CHILLI

Serves 6–8

olive oil
2 red onions, chopped
2 garlic cloves, finely chopped
6 bird's-eye chillies, deseeded and finely chopped
150 g portobello mushrooms, sliced or chopped
1 kg beef mince
2 tins plum tomatoes
2 fresh bay leaves
1 glass red wine
salt
pepper
handful coriander

Heat the oil in a heavy-based pan and cook the onions until soft. Add the garlic, chillies and mushrooms and cook for 5 minutes. Transfer the mixture to a plate and, in the same pan, brown the mince in batches. Add the onion mixture to the beef and then add the tomatoes, bay leaves and red wine. Bring to the boil and simmer for half an hour. Add the kidney beans and simmer for a further half-hour. Season with salt and pepper to taste. Look to cook this long enough to bring it to a thick, 'meaty' consistency, that way it can stand as a substantial 'meal in a bowl' on its own. Stir in the coriander and serve.

SALMON NIÇOISE SALAD (F)
🕐 15 minutes or less
Serves 4

500 g French green beans (haricots verts), topped and tailed
olive oil
salt
pepper
4 salmon fillets – preferably wild or organic
rocket or other salad greens – enough to cover the plate you're using
4 hard-boiled eggs
1/3 of a jar of caper berries

For the dressing
1 clove garlic, finely chopped
1 heaped tsp wholegrain mustard
juice of 2 limes
8 tbsps olive oil
2 tbsps finely chopped parsley

Place the beans in a steamer or pan with a little cold water, and cook until just tender. Toss in olive oil, salt and pepper. Grill fish in a preheated grill for about 5 minutes, turning as necessary. To assemble the salad, use a large platter or plate and cover with the rocket or salad leaves of your choice. Grind some pepper and drizzle a little olive oil over the leaves. Put the beans on top, and arrange the hard-boiled eggs (cut into quarters) around the edge of the platter. Carefully remove the skin from the salmon, break into large chunks and arrange on the salad, or leave whole if you prefer.

Whisk together the dressing ingredients with a fork or put in a clean jam jar and shake. Pour all over the salad and then add the caper berries.

Variations
You may add any other salad vegetables that you like, including cherry tomatoes, strips of red pepper and very thin slithers of fennel. Also, try coriander instead of parsley in the dressing, and scatter a handful of chopped coriander over the whole dish before serving.

VENISON CASSEROLE
olive oil
2 large onions, coarsely chopped
2 sticks of celery, finely chopped
4 carrots, cut into ½-cm discs on a slant
4 cloves of garlic, finely chopped
1 kg venison stewing steak, cut into 2.5-cm chunks and dried on kitchen roll
1/3 bottle of decent red wine
1 can chopped peeled plum tomatoes
2 bay leaves
a couple of sprigs of fresh thyme or a pinch or two of dried
salt
pepper

Pour a generous amount of olive oil into a large, sturdy pot (with a lid). Put on a medium heat. Add the onions and stir occasionally to prevent them from sticking. Add the celery, then the carrots and garlic. While cooking and stirring the vegetables, heat a frying pan with a little olive oil. Brown the venison in batches, transferring to the vegetables as you go along. Once all the meat is browned, add some red wine to this pan and scrape off all the residue on its bottom. Pour the contents of the frying pan and the remainder of the wine over the vegetables and the meat. Then add the tomatoes, the bay leaves and the thyme, and season with salt and pepper. Bring to the boil and cook on a very low simmer for about 3 hours or until the meat is tender, checking from time to time. Alternatively, cook in the oven at about 150°C/300°F/GM2.

Serve on its own or with steamed broccoli, cabbage, green beans or kale.

FRITTATA

⏱ 15 minutes or less
Serves 2–4
A frittata or tortilla, whatever you want to call it, is basically a thick omelette cooked in a non-stick frying pan.

1 large onion, finely chopped
4–6 rashers of good-quality bacon, hard edge of the
rinds removed, cut into 1-cm strips
olive oil
220 g broccoli, cut into small florets
6 medium eggs
salt and pepper

In a non-stick pan, fry the onions and bacon in the oil over a medium heat until cooked. Steam the broccoli for 5 minutes until tender but not soft. Add the broccoli to the onions and bacon in a bowl. Wipe the frying pan clean with some kitchen roll. Beat the eggs in a bowl with some salt and pepper. Put the non-stick frying pan on a medium heat and add olive oil. Add the onions/bacon/broccoli to the eggs and put the whole lot into the heated frying pan.

As the eggs start to cook, using a wooden or heat-resistant plastic spatula, carefully slide the spatula under the eggs and lift so that uncooked mixture can slide underneath. Do this for a minute or so until you feel that the eggs are starting to solidify. When the frittata looks solid enough, take the pan off the heat, give it a shake to make sure that the eggs aren't sticking, and place a large plate over the tortilla. Clamp the plate firmly over the pan and, using oven gloves, carefully but quite swiftly turn the pan upside down so that the frittata ends up on the plate. Put another tablespoon of oil into the pan and slide the frittata back in (what was the top of the frittata should now be face-down in the pan). Gently shake the pan back and forth a few times to ensure the eggs cook evenly and don't stick to the pan. Cook for another 5 minutes or so until cooked through.

If you don't fancy this method, instead of turning the frittata over, you can finish it off under the grill.

This is delicious hot or cold. Serve on its own or with a dressed green salad.

Variations

You can use all sorts of things for the filling, including wilted spinach, roast tomatoes and basil, peas, ham, sautéed courgettes, smoked haddock and so on. Leaving out meat and fish makes this food a good option for vegetarians.

ROAST VEGETABLE AND GOAT'S CHEESE STACK (V)

1 aubergine, sliced into rounds
salt
2 red onions, cut into rings
5 tbsps olive oil
2 tomatoes, skinned and sliced
200 g goat's cheese, sliced

For the marinade
olive oil
1 clove garlic, chopped
4 leaves basil, chopped
salt
pepper

For the sauce
2 shallots, sliced
olive oil
1 tsp tomato purée
1 can chopped tomatoes
water as needed
salt
black pepper

Slice the aubergine, sprinkle with salt and leave for half an hour to allow juices to drain. Wash and pat dry. Place aubergines and onions on a baking tray, lightly brush with oil. Prepare the marinade by mixing the oil, garlic, basil and salt and pepper together. Cover the aubergines, onions and tomatoes in the marinade and leave to rest.

To prepare the sauce, sauté the shallots in a splash of oil until soft, then stir in the tomato purée and canned tomatoes.

Using a hand blender, process the sauce to a smooth consistency, adding a little water to get the right consistency if necessary. Season with salt and pepper and keep warm.

On a baking tray, create four towers by layering the aubergines, tomatoes, onions and goat's cheese slices, then repeat once more, finishing with goat's cheese. Place the tray in a preheated oven at 180°C/350°F/GM4 for 10 to 15 minutes.

To serve, place towers on a pool of sauce on a plate. Serve with a dressed green salad.

BEAN NUT ROAST WITH PEASE PUDDING (V)

230 g adzuki beans, soaked overnight
200 g green lentils, soaked for 1 hour
2 onions, chopped
175 g mixed nuts, chopped
200 g haloumi cheese, grated
1 tbsp chopped parsley
2 eggs, beaten
salt
pepper

For pease pudding
400 g yellow split peas soaked for 1 hour, drained and brought to the boil in fresh water and then simmered for 20–30 minutes until tender, and drained.
1 onion, finely chopped
1 oz butter
1 egg, beaten

To make the nut roast: drain the adzuki beans and bring to boil in the fresh water for 10 minutes. Simmer for 20–30 minutes until tender, then drain. Wash and drain the lentils and bring to the boil in fresh water. Simmer for 20 minutes until tender and drain. Mash the beans and lentils together and mix in the chopped onions. Add the nuts, cheese, parsley and beaten eggs. Season with salt and pepper. Add to a greased and lined loaf tin, and flatten.

To make the pease pudding: grease and line the base of a loaf tin and fill with the drained split peas. Press down firmly and put aside. Fry the onion in butter until soft, add the peas and beaten egg and season. Transfer to a buttered ovenproof dish. Bake the nut roast and pease pudding in a preheated oven 190°C/375°F/GM5 for 30 minutes or until set.

Serve nut roast and pease pudding with vegetables of your choice.

MONKFISH WITH GINGER AND LIME (F)

700 g monkfish, in 2.5-cm chunks
juice of 2 limes
4 cloves garlic, finely chopped
fresh ginger (about a 4-cm length)
olive oil
pepper
salt

Place the monkfish in a bowl large enough to be able to mix the fish with the other ingredients easily. Add the lime juice and chopped garlic. Thinly slice the ginger (a vegetable peeler is ideal for this) into the bowl. Add enough olive oil to coat the fish (about 5 tablespoons), and season with pepper and a little salt. Cover and leave in the fridge for at least 2 hours.

This works very well for a barbecue, in which case remove the monkfish from the marinade and cook for just a few minutes on each side until the fish is cooked through. Otherwise just fry in a little olive oil, or grill.

Serve with a dressed salad and maybe some roast tomatoes.

MACKEREL WITH GARLIC AND ROSEMARY COOKED IN FOIL (F)

whole mackerel
salt
pepper
1 lemon
1 onion
2 cloves garlic, thinly sliced
2 sprigs fresh rosemary
dash of white wine

Preheat the oven to 200°C/400°F/GM6. Put the mackerel in the middle of a large sheet of aluminium foil. Season with salt and pepper. Slice half the lemon and put inside the fish. Juice the remainder of the lemon and pour over the fish. Scatter the onion over the fish, along with the garlic and rosemary. Add the white wine and then wrap the fish up in the foil to make a loose-fitting parcel. Bake in the oven for about 25 minutes.

Serve with dressed salad and/or buttered vegetables.

WOT, NO DESSERTS?

You may have noticed a dearth of desserts here. Desserts by their very nature are sweet, and that generally means the presence of lots of sugar and/or artificial sweeteners, neither of which should assume any prominence in a truly healthy diet. Plus, eating desserts further accustoms the taste buds to sweet foods, which itself can perpetuate a desire for them. In the long run, it can be easier (not to mention healthier) to cut out dessert-eating, apart from on odd occasions, say during a celebratory meal or if you find yourself in a particularly swanky restaurant and simply want to indulge yourself. Any treat of this nature should be savoured and is nothing to feel guilty or regretful about – put eating it in the context of your diet as a whole and see it pale into insignificance.

PRACTICAL POINTS AND SUGGESTIONS

BREAKFAST

I see breakfast as an important meal because, without it, my experience is that very few individuals will be able to make healthy choices easily throughout the rest of the day. There's something about a decent breakfast that seems to 'hold' the appetite in a way that greatly assists healthy eating at lunch and even dinner.

While some people like to eat breakfast at home, this may not always be practical. Some people leave for work too early in the day to make this an option. For this reason it can be good to get into the habit of packing breakfast to have later in the morning. Good breakfast options here include the yoghurt/berries/nuts mix (in a little plastic container – don't forget a spoon), Scotch egg, and even an omelette or frittata. Another option is just to have a few handfuls of nuts (e.g. almonds) and some fruit (e.g. apple). There is nothing wrong with this – just make sure you have enough not to be famished by lunchtime.

My general advice is to make breakfast relatively easy during the week. Something like the yoghurt/berries/ nuts mix or Scotch egg will usually do the trick here. At the weekend, when there's perhaps a bit more time and breakfast is possibly later, that's the time to be a bit more adventurous and branch out into the cooked breakfast, poached eggs and spinach, or scrambled eggs done Indian style. These meals are easier to justify, too, if you're not cooking just for yourself.

If you're away, say in a hotel, then my advice is to opt for a cooked breakfast. Just avoid the bread.

LUNCH

If you're at home, as long as you have the ingredients and a little time, there are plenty of recipes here that will make a good lunch. Examples include the omelette/frittata, sausages and cabbage, and griddled meat (or grilled/fried fish) and tomato/onion/coriander salad. Another option is to reheat something left over from the night before, such as the venison casserole or chilli.

Quick meals also include those where some of the meal is already prepared. For example, reheated Bolognese sauce can be used on top of some freshly cooked cabbage. Or already-prepared home-made burgers can be cooked and placed atop an easily assembled salad.

If you're out of the house at lunch, say at work or elsewhere, then there is an option of packing something. The tuna and bean salad or frittata, for instance, are good options here. Or if there are kitchen facilities at work, then reheated chilli, stir-fry or casserole works well.

If you're eating in a restaurant and are opting for two courses, then something salad-based (e.g. smoked duck salad, or tomato, mozzarella and avocado salad) would be a good place to start. If you're not too hungry, then it's relatively easy to wave away the fancy breads. Follow the salad-based starter with some meat or fish with vegetables (hold the potatoes). If you're vegetarian, opt for something like a roast vegetable stack and salad or just a nice big salad, preferably with some avocado for much-needed protein and fat.

Often the biggest challenge for many lunch-eaters when out of the home is avoiding sandwiches. One alternative is a salad. If you're not vegetarian, I suggest making a conscious effort to getting some meat or fish in you as part of this meal. Many sandwich bars will make up salads or have them already made (e.g. crayfish and avocado salad, falafel salad, chicken Caesar salad). Such eating establishments often offer soups at lunch, usually in the form of both meaty and vegetarian options. If you're not vegetarian, I suggest opting for the meaty varieties as they tend to be more filling and sustaining.

Remember, it's very important not to be too hungry before lunch, as keeping appetite under control really eases the process of making healthy choices. Also bear in mind that what you eat at lunch does not need to get you through to dinner – if you get hungry again, then by all means munch on some nuts or seeds, and perhaps a piece of fruit in the late afternoon or early evening.

TAKEAWAY TAKE-HOME MESSAGES

Takeaway food does not have the healthiest of reputations, and my experience is that individuals admit to eating these with a sense of guilt and remorse. Actually, takeaways do not need to be a nutritional disaster area. It is possible to enjoy them and still eat relatively healthily. The first rule is not to be too hungry when you do the ordering. Grabbing a takeaway late at night while staggering back from the pub with a skinful inside you is not a situation that will lend itself towards healthy food choices.

Ordering a takeaway for you (and perhaps others) on a weekend night in a non-famished state, on the other hand, is much more compatible with healthy eating. The trick is to think 'primal'. So, if Indian food is the order of the day, opt for a meat- or prawn-based curry, or tikka dish, plus vegetables, say in the form of sag paneer (Indian cheese and spinach) and dahl (lentils). If you're not too hungry, you won't miss the rice and nan that really do the damage. If Chinese food is in the offing, opt maybe for a beef, prawn or chicken dish (e.g. beef with ginger, spicy prawns, chicken with cashew nuts) and some stir-fried vegetables. Hold the rice.

Oh, and if you do happen to find yourself hungry in the dead of night and in need of some immediate stomach satisfaction, my advice is to seek out a shish kebab – unadulterated lamb, raw vegetables and not too much in the way of an unhealthy carb load (bread) won't do much harm in the grand scheme of things.

DINNER

In comparison to breakfast and lunch, dinner is generally easier to manage. In a restaurant, I would follow the advice offered above for lunchtime (salad starter, followed by meat/fish and vegetables or vegetarian salad). The same goes for room service. At home, options are generally much broader (see Meals recipes, above).

Some people are concerned about eating too late at night. Personally, I think the real problem is not eating too late, it's eating *too much* too late. There's an argument for eating smaller evening meals than we traditionally do. Appetite control is key here, so eating well during the day and grabbing a snack in the late afternoon/early evening can be critical.

It's a good idea to get into the habit of seeing dinner as a generally one-course meal (unless, of course it's a special occasion, dinner party, etc). A bowl of seafood stew or chilli, for instance, should suffice as long as your appetite has not been allowed to run out of control.

Alcohol can be an issue for some in the evening. Some suggestions regarding this were made in the last chapter (Liquid Assets). In brief, make sure you're not too hungry or thirsty in the evening, and match each alcoholic drink with a glass of water.

SNACKS

One central tenet of the advice in *Waist Disposal* is the avoidance of undue hunger, and snacking can most certainly have a part to play here. While fruit is often hailed as the snack of choice, I disagree. The problem with fruit is that, while generally healthy, it can often do little or nothing in terms of sating the appetite, and therefore will not tide you over nicely till dinner.

A much better option, I think, would be nuts (preferably in their raw form). Many people find that raw almonds work for them, though other alternatives obviously exist (e.g. walnuts, pecans, cashews). Some of the other attributes of nuts are that they are generally readily available, are convenient to carry around or store in a desk, and keep well.

Other than nuts, foods that make good snacks for those seeking to control their hunger are hard-boiled eggs, Scotch eggs, olives, biltong (dried meat) and cold meats (e.g. roast beef, cold chicken).

Sometimes we have occasion to sit down for a slightly more substantial snack, maybe at the weekend. Let's say you've had a large cooked breakfast late in the morning, and don't want a full lunch but do need something reasonably substantial to get you comfortably through to dinner. A plate of cheese and celery may fit the bill here, and this could also be coupled with some cold/cooked meats and olives.

GET READY FOR READY-MEALS

There's a strong theme in these recommendations: your diet should be made up, as much as possible, of natural, unprocessed foods. However, we don't always have the time to cook foods from fresh ingredients, and this is one reason why some of us may be tempted by convenience foods and ready-meals. At lot of these, for example microwaveable lasagne, are never going to get you closer to your fat-loss and health goals. However, that does not mean to say that all ready-meals are off-limits.

A ready-meal made up of a piece of fish or meat accompanied by some vegetables is, to all intents and purposes, no more processed that something you might prepare at home. Yes, it might have a bit more salt than you would use, but it's essentially quite unprocessed. As with takeaways, the trick is to stick to ready-meals that are made from 'primal' ingredients. Such meals are a good compromise between healthy eating and convenience.

SAMPLE EATING PLANS

What follows are some examples of what a typical day's eating might look like for you. The weekday options have some emphasis on ease and practicality (particularly at breakfast). The weekend options are based on somewhat more substantial breakfasts, and more ambitious evening meals, too. The snacks are optional – if you don't need them to keep your appetite under control, don't eat them.

These are obviously only sample eating plans, used to demonstrate how putting together the dietary suggestions here might look in the real world. These plans can be used to inspire your own choices, based on your own food preferences.

WEEKDAY OPTIONS

Breakfast: yoghurt, nut and berry mix
Snack: raw almonds
Lunch: crayfish and avocado salad (bought)
Snack: raw almonds and some dark chocolate
Dinner: home-made beefburger and salad

Breakfast: 1–2 Scotch eggs
Snack: raw mixed nuts
Lunch: tuna and bean salad or reheated chilli
Snack: mixed nuts and a piece of fruit (e.g. apple or pear)
Dinner: grilled salmon with tomato, onion and coriander salad

Breakfast: chorizo and goat's cheese omelette (either hot or cold)
Snack: raw almonds
Lunch: meaty soup (bought)
Snack: raw almonds and some dark chocolate
Dinner: monkfish with lime and salad

WEEKEND OPTIONS

Breakfast/brunch: cooked breakfast
Snack: raw almonds and piece of fruit
Lunch/snack: cheese, celery and cold meats
Dinner: venison casserole and vegetables

Breakfast/brunch: scrambled eggs, Indian style
Snack: raw almonds and piece of fruit
Lunch: cheese, celery and cold meats
Snack: raw mixed nuts
Dinner: venison casserole and vegetables

Breakfast/brunch: scrambled eggs with smoked salmon
Snack: raw almonds
Lunch: tuna and egg salad
Snack: raw mixed nuts and dark chocolate
Dinner: roast chicken with Piri Piri sauce

Chapter 10

MUSCLE BOUND

HOW TO GET FIT AND TONED IN JUST 12 MINUTES A DAY

For you, a likely motivation for reading this book and putting its advice into action is a desire to turn a somewhat flabby, out-of-condition body into a slimmer, more athletic one. There are two main approaches to sculpting the body of your dreams: losing fat, and building and toning muscle. The former has been the focus of this book thus far. This chapter is about the latter.

In this chapter you'll be introduced to a regime of exercises designed to bring significant results, in terms of improving the look and strength of your body, in just 12 minutes a day. This regime is based on what is known as 'resistance' exercise – the form of exercise essential for building and strengthening muscle. More about this later.

The other major type of exercise is termed 'aerobic' exercise, examples of which include running, cycling and rowing. Regular aerobic exercise is advocated for its benefits on health including, a reduced risk of heart disease and type 2 diabetes, and is believed to have mood-enhancing effects, too.

'Exercise more' is a core piece of advice for individuals wanting to lose weight. Just like the 'eat less' mantra, this advice appears eminently sensible at first glance: if body weight is determined by the amount of calories we expend relative to the amount we take in, then surely expending more calories must lead to weight loss? However, as we learned in Chapter 2 (The Calorie Trap), eating less might not be effective for long-term weight loss. Could the same be true for exercising more?

DOES AEROBIC EXERCISE PROMOTE WEIGHT LOSS?

Imagine for a moment that you're carrying a bit of a spare tyre and are committed to taking exercise to get rid of it. Let's say you decide to take up jogging, and start taking the oft-quoted advice to get through 30 minutes of exercise, five times a week. A 30-minute jog will burn about 290 calories. However, just sitting watching television will burn about 40 calories in the same time, so the additional calorie burn for half an hour's worth of jogging is 250 calories. The total calorie burn from exercise for the week comes to 1,250 calories (250 x 5). Now, assuming that all of those calories will be lost in the form of fat, and that you don't eat a bit more as a result of expending more energy (more on this in a moment), then the amount of fat lost over the week from your jogging endeavours is about 140 g (less than a third of a pound).

Compare this to the theoretical calorie deficit that can be achieved through a change in diet. When individuals go from a carb-loaded diet to one lower in carb and higher in protein, there is usually an automatic reduction in calorie intake because the latter diet is more satisfying. In one study, such a swap led to a spontaneous reduction in intake of about 1,000 calories a day.[1] Let's imagine, though, that as a result of changing your diet you eat, say, 500 fewer calories each day without feeling hungry. Total calorie deficit for the week would be 3,500 calories, which equates to one pound of fat. In other words, the dietary intervention produces three times the results achieved by jogging, and with far less physical effort, too.

Some claim that additional calories are burned *after* exercise, too; this needs to be factored into our assessment. The idea that exercise promotes fat-burning is true. However, the effect is relatively small, and unlikely to lead to any meaningful weight loss. The most recent evidence in this area has shown that, for moderate-intensity activities lasting up to an hour in length, fat metabolism over the next 24 hours is essentially the same as it would have been if no exercise had been taken.[2]

Exercise is not a particularly effective way of burning calories and fat. And there's another thing that you should know about exercise if you're planning to use it to lose weight ...

EXERCISE CAN WORK UP AN APPETITE

People who exercise more tend to be hungrier and eat more, too.[3] Undoing the calorie deficit induced by a 30-minute jog doesn't take much, either (three plain digestive biscuits will do it). Many people find that stepping up their exercise leads quite naturally to an increase in food intake. This phenomenon, coupled with the fact that reasonable levels of exercise don't burn many calories, might make achieving a significant calorie deficit through exercise well-nigh impossible.

WHAT DOES THE SCIENCE SHOW?

Theoretically, exercise does not look like a particularly efficient or viable way of losing weight. But what does the science show? Has exercise been found to be beneficial for those seeking to shed excess pounds, or not?

The most comprehensive assessment of the impact of exercise on weight loss to date was conducted by members of an international group of independent researchers known as the Cochrane Collaboration. The review included 43 individual studies, and its point was to quantify the effect that exercise has on weight loss.[4] The amount of exercise prescribed in these studies varied from study to study. Typically, exercise sessions lasted 45 minutes with a frequency of three to five times a week. The total length of the studies ranged between 3 and 12 months.

The individual studies in this review were designed to study different things. For instance, some of them compared the impact of exercise or diet on weight loss. Here the results showed that the 'dieters' lost between 2.8 kg and 13.6 kg in weight. On the other hand, exercisers lost between just 0.5 and 4.0 kg in weight. In other words, dietary change is far more effective than exercise in bringing about weight loss.

Some other studies in this review compared the effect of diet and exercise with dietary change alone. Here it was found that weight loss for those dieting and exercising was between 3.4 and 17.7 kg, but for those just dieting it was 2.3–16.7 kg.

Overall, the additional weight loss from exercise averaged out at a shade over 1 kg.

Imagine cleaning up your diet and in six months you find you've lost 10 kg in weight. If, on top of this, you had been exercising for 45 minutes, four times a week, you could expect to have lost about 11 kg. And the time you would have spent exercising to get this additional 1 kg weight loss benefit? *69 hours.*

What all this means is that if you've already made a commitment to dietary change, then exercising for, say, several hours each week is likely to have little or no additional effect on your weight-loss efforts.

This is not to say that aerobic exercise is a waste of time – it most certainly is not. The science links exercise with improvements in health and reduced risk of chronic disease (see below).

But, the science also shows that exercise, generally speaking, is not effective for the purposes of weight loss per se.

COULD POOR WEIGHT-LOSS RESULTS FROM EXERCISE BE DOWN TO MUSCLE GAIN?

One explanation for the failure of exercise to induce weight loss could be this: exercisers build muscle, which offsets the weight that is lost due to fat melting away. The thing is, though, the exercises deployed in the studies reviewed above were 'aerobic' activities that don't build muscle. The logical conclusion is, therefore, that aerobic exercise is quite ineffective for weight and fat loss.

WHAT ABOUT WEIGHT MAINTENANCE?

Exercise, overall, is not effective for weight loss, but could it help with weight maintenance? Once you've shed the required amount of flab, could exercise help you maintain your leaner condition? The answer to this appears to be 'yes', but the best available evidence suggests that exercise is, again, not a particularly efficient or effective way of going about it.

For example, one study[5] found that exercise slowed (but didn't stop) weight regain at a rate of 50 g (1.76 oz) per month (not much). The evidence suggests that successful maintenance of weight loss through exercise requires a considerable amount of time and effort: one major review found that 60–90 minutes of daily activity is required to increase substantially someone's chances of preventing weight regain after weight loss.[6] That's a lot of time spent exercising just to stand still from a weight perspective.

WHAT'S THE POINT OF AEROBIC EXERCISE, THEN?

All this talk about how ineffective exercise generally is for weight loss and weight maintenance may give you the impression that I'm somewhat anti-exercise. I most certainly am not. I am, however, not keen to perpetuate a commonly-held myth about the value of aerobic exercise in shedding pounds.

I am genuinely enthusiastic about exercise, because while it may not help much with weight loss, it is linked with a reduced risk of a variety of conditions including heart disease and type 2 diabetes, and is associated with a reduced risk of death, too. In addition, regular activity appears to have a natural mood-enhancing and anti-depressant activity. So, regular aerobic activity is to be recommended most heartily.

One form of aerobic exercise that I think has particular merit is walking. Some people take the view that walking is not strenuous enough to benefit health and fitness. The evidence suggests otherwise.

For example, in one study[7] individuals were instructed to walk briskly for a total of 30 minutes, three or five times a week. Individuals could break down the 30 minutes into periods of no fewer than 10 minutes. Other individuals in this study were not given any walking instructions, and therefore acted as a 'control' or 'inactive' group against whom the results of the 'walkers' could be compared. The research was conducted over a 12-week period.

The researchers involved in this study assessed the participants with a number of measurements which included blood pressure, waist and hip circumference, and functional capacity (fitness). Systolic blood pressure (the higher value of the blood-pressure measurement) fell significantly in both the three- and five-times-a-week walkers. Plus, fitness increased in both groups, too.

There was one other notable benefit from exercise: Waist circumference fell significantly in those who were taking exercise (about an inch in both groups). Remember, all these benefits can come from nothing more strenuous than walking.

In 2007, an editorial published in the *British Medical Journal* reviewed the evidence regarding the benefits of walking.[8] The review pointed to evidence which shows that greater walking distances and speed are associated with lower risk of cardiovascular disease, type 2 diabetes, and overall risk of death.[9,10] The risk in the most active walkers was about half that of those who were least active.

TAKING EXERCISE OUTSIDE IN THE SUN MAY HAVE PARTICULAR BENEFITS

One great thing about walking is that it gives us a good excuse to get outside. This opens up the possibility of spin-off benefits from walking or other outdoor pursuits that have nothing to do with exercise *per se*. What I'm referring to here are the myriad health benefits to be had from exposure to sunlight.

For example, in the winter, low levels of sun exposure can lead to suppressed mood and even depression (seasonal affective disorder). This can be combated by, obviously, getting ourselves into the light.

Sunlight, particularly in the warmer months, can boost vitamin D levels in the body. Higher levels of this nutrient appear to protect against a dizzying array of conditions including cardiovascular disease, several forms of cancer, diabetes, multiple sclerosis and bone disease. Enhanced vitamin D levels are also associated with a reduced risk of death.

Vitamin D may also help you in your activity and exercise endeavours. It plays a part in the formation of muscle, and appears to enhance fitness, too. One study reviewed evidence for the ability of vitamin D to enhance athletic performance.[11] The review cites studies in which vitamin D supplementation was found to increase measures of type 2 (fast twitch) muscle fibres, *without any physical training*.

The review also cited evidence which links higher vitamin D levels in the body with improved muscular strength, balance, reaction time and physical performance. The authors of this review went back to old research in which researchers assessed the impact of ultraviolet (UV) light treatment (which has the capacity to raise vitamin D levels) on physical performance. For example, in the 1940s, German researchers treated adults with UV light twice a week for six weeks. Performance on a stationary bicycle increased by 13 per cent. However, in non-treated individuals, performance was unchanged.

In another study from the same time, UV treatment was tested in a group of college students undergoing physical training. Physical fitness increased by more than 19 per cent in these students, compared to a similarly-trained group not exposed to UV light therapy.

Another study cited by the authors examined the effect of UV therapy on children. UV lights were installed in the classroom of 120 schoolchildren and used for nine months of the year. After this, fitness was assessed using a stationary bicycle. Compared to children who had not undergone UV therapy, treated children were a quite amazing 56 per cent fitter.

The evidence suggests that simply sitting in the sun can make us fitter, healthier and happier.

EXERCISE INTENSITY

It is generally accepted that exercise needs to be of a certain intensity to get any meaningful benefit from it. Intensity of exercise can be expressed as a percentage of the maximum heart rate a person is capable of. A decent guide to your maximum heart rate is 220 minus your age.

Generally speaking, exercising at about 50–70 per cent of maximum heart rate is considered enough to help someone attain or maintain fitness, and is also a level of intensity that is likely to give someone the health-enhancing and disease-protective benefits exercise can bestow. To attain even the upper end of this intensity spectrum doesn't necessarily take too much effort. Many individuals will be able to achieve a pulse rate of 70 per cent maximum heart rate just by walking.

If you're unfit and out of condition and carrying a lot of extra fat, you won't necessarily need to walk that quickly to get up to 70 per cent of your maximum heart rate. If you're in good condition, though, there's still a good chance that walking will get you up there as long as the walk you're taking is genuinely *brisk*.

If you're not going to check your pulse or use a heart-rate monitor, then aim for a level of intensity where you are somewhat breathless but still able to conduct a conversation. If you can sing (should you want to), you're probably not working hard enough.

The evidence strongly suggests that walking has the power to boost health and fitness. It has other things going for it too, namely:

1. **Almost everyone can do it, and you don't need to be particularly 'sporty' to do it, either.**

2. **Even at relatively high intensity, walking tends to be gentle on the joints and muscles and has low risk of injury.**

3. **It doesn't require any special equipment, and can often be incorporated quite naturally during the day (weather conditions permitting).**

HOW MUCH IS ENOUGH?

The evidence on how much exercise is required to get significant benefits for health is mixed, but there is good reason to believe that 30 minutes a day on most days of the week is likely to reap long-term benefits.

Something that can put people off exercise is the thought that they are not going to be able to spare half an hour for walking or other form of exercise. However, if truth be told, many of us could liberate 30 minutes of each day quite easily. Here are a few suggestions for how:

- **Don't turn on the television in the evening (or any other time of day, for that matter).**

- **Get up earlier (getting to bed a bit earlier is the secret here).**

- Avoid checking and reading emails incessantly: aim for 1–3 checks at predetermined times each day. If required, set an auto-responder detailing the times you will be checking emails, and how you can be contacted if something is *really* urgent.
- Don't buy a newspaper – very rarely is anything important going to be missed by not getting one's daily fix of print media.
- Schedule exercise into the day – at the start of every day or week, work out where your activity is going to go, put it in your diary and commit to it as you would a meeting or appointment.

Just employing one or two of these strategies will usually be all it takes to free up the time to weave some walking or other form of exercise into your life with relative ease.

But what if you really can't find a straight half-hour for some exercise, what then?

IS IT OK TO SPLIT EXERCISE UP?

Some studies have explored whether the benefits of exercise remain if, say, a continuous 30-minute bout of exercise is split up into smaller chunks. The good news is the results of these studies suggest that the benefits are just the same. For example, in one study, three 10-minute bouts of exercise a day led to the same improvements in blood fat (triglyceride) and blood-pressure levels as a continuous 30-minute bout of walking.[12]

In another study, women exercised for a total of 30 minutes each day, several times each week. For some women this 30 minutes was made up of one continuous session; for others it was made up of two 15-minute sessions over the course of the day; for still others, it was divided into three 10-minute sessions. All three groups saw similar improvement in measures of fitness.[13]

IF YOU WANT TO STEP UP YOUR WALKING, BUY A PEDOMETER

Pedometers are small, usually inexpensive, battery-operated devices that are worn on the belt and count your steps. Evidence suggests that wearing one of these helps people to be more active. In one piece of research, scientists reviewed the relationship between pedometer use and activity levels, with two types of evidence: 'observational studies' (where activity levels were compared in pedometer users and non-users in a population) and 'randomised controlled trials' (where some individuals where instructed to use a pedometer and others were not).[14]

The results showed that pedometer use was associated with greater walking distances (about an additional 2,500 steps per day). Overall, pedometer use was associated with about a 27 per cent increase in physical activity.

What is also interesting about this study is that it found that increased activity was especially likely in individuals who had a goal of walking at least a set number of steps a day.

Overall, the results of this research suggest that investing in a pedometer and having a daily stepping target might help to motivate individuals to be more active over time.

OFFER SOME RESISTANCE

Apart from aerobic exercise such as walking, the other major form of exercise is known as 'resistance exercise'. As its name suggests, this form of exercise uses significant resistance to a force generated by contracting muscles.

Lifting weights is an example of this. However, some resistance exercises effectively use the body as the 'weight' that creates resistance. A press-up, for example, uses the body as a weight against which certain muscles (e.g. the triceps and chest muscles) push.

Resistance exercise is distinct from aerobic exercises such as jogging and swimming in that it's generally harder work, and is therefore something that cannot be maintained for extended periods of time. On the plus side, the intensity of resistance exercise is what gives it the potential to improve the size and tone of muscles in a way aerobic exercise simply can't. Resistance exercise can transform the look of the body, as well as enhance muscular strength.

DOES MUSCLE-BUILDING BOOST THE METABOLISM?

Earlier on we learned that aerobic exercise is not particularly effective at boosting fat-burning. However, because muscle is more 'metabolically active' than fat, could losing fat and building muscle allow us to burn calories 'for free' even when we are sitting on our bums watching telly or surfing the internet? What sort of advantage can we expect here?

Let's do some maths. A kilogram of fat burns about 4.5 calories a day (not very much). A kilogram of muscle at rest burns about 13 calories a day (much more than fat, but still not very much). Now, imagine you lose a kg of fat and gain a kg of muscle, then the additional benefit in terms of calorie burning, theoretically anyway, is 8.5 calories a day. Over a year, that would amount to a benefit of about 3,100 calories. There's 9 calories in a gram of fat, so assuming all this benefit translated into a loss of fat (which is not assured, at all), the amount of fat lost is about 350 grams or ¾ of a pound. Even when we, say, multiply the numbers by 5 (5 kg of fat loss, 5 kg of muscle gained) the theoretical advantage is still small. And this is assuming, by the way, that the increased exercise required to build muscle and its greater metabolic activity does not somehow drive us to eat more.

While exercise (whether aerobic or resistance in form) is an ineffective and inefficient way to lose fat, there are still significant advantages to building or maintaining muscle. For a start, when you're losing weight, there's the risk that some of this will come from muscle. Resistance exercise reduces the risk of this happening.

In one study, individuals were put on a calorie-restricted diet. The group was then divided into three. One group engaged in resistance exercise, one group engaged in aerobic exercise, and the other group just dieted. All groups lost the same amount of weight (more evidence that exercise does not assist weight loss), though the resistance-training group lost significantly less muscle.[15]

The role of diet in maintaining muscle mass was reviewed by scientists from the University of Westminster, London.[16] In this review the authors highlight the role of resistance training for preserving muscle mass. They also, by the way, reiterate the point that consuming adequate amounts of protein plays a key role here, too.

Another reason for doing resistance exercise is that it can improve strength. It's never a bad thing in life to be able to lift heavy boxes and luggage with relative ease, and maybe win the odd arm-wrestling contest, too. But muscle strength seems to have other important implications as well, in that it is associated with a reduced risk of premature death. A study published in the *British Medical Journal* assessed the relationship between muscular strength and the risk of mortality in 9,000 men aged 20–80.[17] Muscular strength was assessed using leg- and bench-presses. The men were then divided into three categories of strength: lower, middle and upper. The men were followed up for almost 19 years.

The risk of mortality (overall risk of death) was then compared across the groups, having adjusted for a number of confounding factors such as age, fitness, smoking, medical history and family history of cardiovascular disease. Compared to those in the 'lower' strength category, those in the 'middle' and 'upper' strength categories were found to be at a significantly reduced risk of death.

Of course, another reason for working your muscles is to get them – and you – looking better. If the last time you did a press-up was in a singlet and plimsolls in your school gym, then there's a good chance your muscles will be somewhat flaccid and lacking in shape and tone. Even if you lose fat, you may still end up with a body that looks a bit limp and, frankly, unappealing. That's where resistance exercise comes in.

A COMPLETE WORKOUT IN 12 MINUTES

Some people tense up simply on hearing the expression 'resistance exercise'. Why? Maybe because it conjures up images of bodybuilders with over developed musculature lifting eye-popping weights. Relax. Building a stronger body and better-looking physique doesn't have to be this way, or anything close.

It is possible to improve the look and condition of the body significantly, quite quickly and easily and with relatively low time-investment, too. What we have here is a 12-minute daily programme that is mainly resistance-exercise based, but includes some aerobic exercise, too. It can be performed in a space no bigger than a beach towel and requires little or no special equipment. If you do nothing other than this 12-minute routine each day, you will still be able to improve your strength and physique to a significant and tangible extent.

The session is actually made up of two six-minute sections. The first six minutes focus on resistance exercises for the upper body. The second six minutes are designed to work the legs with both resistance and aerobic exercise.

SPECIAL EQUIPMENT

There are really only two pieces of equipment you need to consider purchasing:

1. Dyna-Band or something similar

Dyna-Bands are essentially large, wide, coloured elastic bands, a few feet in length. They can be useful for performing certain exercises including biceps curls and one-armed rows (see below). They come in different colours, each of which denotes a different resistance. One of the great things about this exercise aid is that it is small and light, and therefore perfect for people who travel or are on the road a lot and want to maintain their exercise regime, wherever they are.

2. Dumbbells

A set of dumbbells can be a great investment. Go for a set where the amount of weight can be varied. These are obviously not for packing in your hand luggage, but a great piece of equipment if you're planning on exercising at home.

THE FIRST SIX MINUTES

The first six minutes of the session are divided into one-minute blocks, each of which is designed to work a major muscle or muscle group. These are:

1. Chest

2. Back

3. Shoulders

4. Biceps

5. Triceps

6. Abdominals

HOW HARD SHOULD I WORK?

Your ultimate aim is to keep consistent 'form' for each exercise for the whole minute. At the same time, at the end of the minute you should be struggling to perform additional repetitions. Adjust the dumbbell weight or tension in the Dyna-Band (if relevant), as well as the speed of repetitions, accordingly. As you progress, you can increase these variables to add to your workload.

Full press-ups (see below) are quite hard to do. You may want to start with less intensive versions of this exercise (half press-up or box press-up) to begin with, graduating to full press-ups in time if this is appropriate.

1. CHEST
Press-ups

Press-ups exercise and strengthen several muscles including the pectoral muscles (chest) and triceps (at the back of the upper arm). They also work muscles at the side of the chest wall and in the back.

There's a choice of three here:

- **Full press-up – keep your hips and knees straight. Your hands should be directly under your shoulders. Lower your body by bending your elbows until your chest is** about 10 cm from the floor. Push up again. In addition to exercising the muscles listed above, full press-ups count as a 'core stability' exercise – meaning that it helps strengthen muscles in and around the abdomen, lower back and pelvis.

- Half press-up – similar to full press-ups, but the knees are on the ground set behind the hips.

- Box press-up – similar to the half, but the knees are directly under the hips.

2. BACK
One-armed Rows

This exercise is designed to work muscles in the back, principally *lattimus dorsi* (seen most prominently adjacent to the upper arms) and the rhomboids (which run from the inner shoulder blade to the spine). It also exercises the upper arm.

To perform a one-armed row, stand left side-on to a sofa or bed and put your left knee on the sofa/bed. Lean forward and put your left hand on the sofa/bed. Keep your right foot on the floor. Trap the Dyna-Band under your right foot and hold the end in your right hand (or alternatively hold a dumbbell in your right hand). Pull your right hand up to your upper chest, hold briefly and then relax. This exercise is for the right side of the back. The active part of this exercise is essentially the same as the action used to start petrol lawnmowers with a cord starter.

Reverse the position (right hand and knee on sofa/bed, left hand holding the Dyna-Band/dumbbell) to exercise the left side of your back.

3. SHOULDERS
Shoulder Presses

The shoulder press principally works the deltoid muscles, which are the major muscles in the shoulders at the top of the arms.

To perform the shoulder press, sit comfortably in a firm chair with your back straight. Take dumbbells in both hands and hold in front of your chest with your thumbs pointing towards your chest. Lift the dumbbells above your head, pause briefly, and return the dumbbells in a controlled fashion to the front of your chest.

This exercise can be performed using a Dyna-Band. Sit on the Dyna-Band and take the ends in each hand. Alternatively you can perform the exercise while standing with the Dyna-Band trapped under both your feet. You may need to tie two Dyna-Bands together to make it long enough.

4. BICEPS
Biceps Curls
The biceps is the major muscle at the front of the upper arm.

To perform biceps curls, stand with dumbbells in each hand and let your arms hang, palms facing forward. Lift both dumbbells to your shoulders, pause briefly and lower again in a controlled fashion.

This exercise can be performed using a Dyna-Band, in which case the Dyna-Band should be trapped under both feet.

5. TRICEPS
Triceps Dips
The triceps is the major muscle at the back of the upper arm. You will need a chair for this exercise. Place the front of the chair behind you. Put your palms on the seat of the chair with your fingers pointing forward. Bend your knees and keep your feet flat on the floor. Take your weight on your arms and slowly bend your elbows to 90 degrees, lowering your hips towards the floor. Push back up again. Keep your back straight and close to the chair throughout this exercise.

If, on occasion, you do not have access to a chair or something similar and are unable to perform this exercise, don't worry – press-ups (see above) will give your triceps a decent workout.

6. ABDOMINALS
Sit-ups
Lie with your back flat on the floor, knees bent and feet flat. Place your right hand on your right thigh and place your left hand behind your neck. Slowly lift your left shoulder off the floor by squeezing your abdominal muscles. Curl your upper torso as you move forward towards your knees. Slide your hand along your thigh until your wrist gets to your knee. Hold briefly, and lower yourself back to the ground slowly and in a controlled fashion. Keep your lower back in contact with the floor throughout this exercise, and do not pull your neck or head with the supporting hand. Repeat on the other side.

START SLOWLY
The aim with these exercises is to do them continuously for a minute (or as long as you can reasonably manage). If you are out of condition and new to resistance exercise, then start with relatively low loads. Choose your Dyna-Band resistance and vary the length of slack accordingly. With the dumbbells, start with relatively light weights and build up over time. With press-ups, perhaps opt for the half- or box-type first, before graduating to the full form. With the triceps dips, maybe start by not going all the way down.

Once you're through with these upper-body exercises, it's time to work on your legs.

THE SECOND SIX MINUTES

The second six minutes are a combination of jogging on the spot (aerobic) with resistance exercise for the legs, in the form of squats.

1. Jogging on the Spot

The aim here is not to leap and bound away, but to take relatively small steps, lifting your feet about 10 cm off the floor.

Jogging on the spot may be too intense an exercise to maintain for six minutes for some. An alternative would be to march on the spot, in which case the legs should be raised about 30 cm off the floor. As you get fitter you may want to introduce jogging on the spot gradually into the regime until, ultimately, you're able to jog on the spot throughout.

2. Squats

Place your feet a little more than shoulder-width apart, toes pointed out slightly. Sit back until your thighs are roughly parallel with the floor (the hips should end up higher than the knees). Keep your knees over your ankles and swing your arms forward as you sit back, to keep your balance. Return to standing and repeat.

Start the second six-minute session by running on the spot for 75 counts where you count each time your left foot hits the floor (one count equals one step with each foot). After this, immediately perform 10 squats. Repeat this sequence until six minutes have elapsed. Depending on your fitness, you should get through 450–675 steps in six minutes.

That's it!

This 12-minute regime provides a great resistance workout for the upper and lower body, with some aerobic conditioning thrown in. All in the comfort of your own home or hotel room, with no special gear or equipment required save a giant rubber band or pair of dumbbells.

HOW OFTEN SHOULD I DO THIS?

There is a notion in muscle-building that, after being worked, muscles need time to repair, and it's during repair that muscles grow and get stronger. This has led to the idea that no muscle group should be exercised more than about once or twice a week. This advice usually refers to exercises where a single muscle group may have been the focus of someone's attention in the gym for perhaps an hour or more. In this time, serious damage may be induced. No wonder it takes a week or so for that damage to be repaired.

The damage induced by this 12-minute session will be minor in comparison. Each muscle group is only engaged for a minute each time, and at loads that are worthwhile, but do not cause 'failure' (when you simply can't do another repetition). The recommended intensity is certainly enough to make real progress, but not enough to require days for recovery.

When you first start this programme, if you haven't done much for a while, then you may well be a bit sore the following day and perhaps for another day or two. At the outset, let soreness be your guide as to when to next do the session. Once your muscles have little detectable soreness, you're good to go again. In the beginning, this may mean resting for two or more days between sessions. But the fitter and stronger you get, the quicker your recovery will be. Ultimately, you should be able to do the session every day, with no soreness in between sessions.

LOW-CARBOHYDRATE DIETS AND EXERCISE

Some of you may be familiar with the concept of 'carb-loading'. The idea is that during exercise that has some aerobic component (e.g. football, rugby, running, cycling), much of the body's fuel comes from glycogen (a carbohydrate) stored in the liver and muscles. Prior to sport, then, it is often advised that plenty of carbs are eaten to fill up the glycogen stores so that plenty of ready energy will be available during exercise. So, theoretically, a low-carbohydrate diet could lead to depleted glycogen stores, and impaired performance.

Let's work through some figures. As we explored earlier, a 30-minute jog will burn about 250 additional calories. A significant proportion of the fuel for this exercise will come from fat. Let's imagine that, during the jog, 150 of the calories come from carb. Each gram of carbohydrate contains 4 calories, so in theory to replenish the glycogen lost during exercise you are going to need to consume about 40 grams of carb. That's about the same amount of carb found in a couple of apples.

In other words, for most individuals engaged in recreational exercise that doesn't go on for hours, glycogen depletion is unlikely to be an issue unless carb consumption is cut to very low levels.

For endurance sports, low-carb eating is potentially more of an issue. If you're training for a marathon, for instance, and racking up 50 miles or more a week, then glycogen depletion is a real risk. However, one thing that needs to be borne in mind is that when carbohydrate is restricted, the body automatically turns to other fuels (principally fat) to make up the difference.

This adaptation can take time, so adopting a low-carb diet is not the thing to do a week before a marathon, particularly if your goal is not just to 'get round' but to crack your personal best.

At lower intensities of exercise, however, adopting a low-carbohydrate diet does not appear to be an impediment to activity. A major review on the subject concluded that '… endurance performance can be sustained despite the virtual exclusion of carbohydrate from the human diet.'[18]

There is no doubt in my mind that the very physically active can tolerate more carb in their diet than those who are not. If this applies to you, then aim to get your additional carbohydrate into the system within an hour or so after a sporting event or training session (this helps replenish glycogen in the muscles for future use).

If you do feel the need to do this, I would counsel against using bread, pasta and white rice as your carbohydrate sources. Not only are these foods generally disruptive to blood sugar, they also offer precious little from a nutritional perspective. As we explored in Chapter 3, this sort of fare is not so much food, as *fodder*. Generally, slower sugar-releasing and more nutritious forms of carbohydrate include fruit, vegetables and legumes (beans and lentils).

BACK TO BASICS

- Exercise is often promoted as a way to lose weight.
- Generally speaking, exercise burns relatively few calories.
- People who exercise more, tend to eat more, too.

- It's difficult to induce a calorie deficit through exercise.

- Studies show that exercise is not an efficient or effective way to lose weight.

- Aerobic exercise may not help weight loss, but is associated with a range of benefits for health including a reduced risk of cardiovascular disease and type 2 diabetes, and improved mood.

- Walking has been found to confer significant health benefits.

- Aim to walk for a total of 30 minutes on most days of the week.

- Research shows that the benefits of exercise still exist if performed as multiple, short-duration sessions.

- Resistance exercise can build and tone muscle, improving body composition as well as strength and the look of the body.

- Considerable improvements in these factors can be had by exercising for as little as 12 minutes a day.

Chapter 11

MIND MATTERS

HOW TO HARNESS THE POWER OF YOUR MIND TO TRANSFORM YOUR BODY

The brain has an overarching influence on all bodily actions and processes. From the regulation of the body's internal environment, to physical actions such as walking, talking, eating and drinking, the brain acts as central HQ. In recent years there has been growing recognition that our thoughts can have a profound influence on how our body functions. Certain emotions, for example aggression and hostility, have been linked with negative effects on the body, including an increased risk of heart disease and impairment of the immune system. But there's another side to this: certain beliefs and thought processes may positively affect health and wellbeing. This chapter is about how you can use your mind to accelerate the transformation of your body into something trimmer and more toned.

YOU BETTER BELIEVE IT

One of the most startling examples of the power of the mind to influence health is the placebo response. For example, give individuals in pain a dummy pill (placebo) but tell them it's a painkiller, and a third or more of them will get significant pain-relief from it. The same is true for depressed individuals given dummy pills dressed up as antidepressants. Clearly, the mind has the capacity to induce considerable self-healing – if the mental conditions are right.

Could the same be true for, say, weight loss or fitness? Could a change in thinking have benefits here?

This was the question that was essentially posed in a study published in 2007.[1] In this piece of research, 84 hotel chambermaids were split into two groups. One group was told that their work constituted good exercise and satisfied the official recommendations for maintaining health and fitness. To reinforce this message, the group was given examples of how their work-related activity supposedly constituted decent exercise. The other group, on the other hand, were told nothing.

The women were monitored over a four-week period, during which activity levels stayed the same in the two groups. However, the group who had been told their work constituted good exercise *believed* they were getting more exercise than before. And, compared to the other group, these women saw a reduction in blood pressure, weight, body fat percentage and waist-to-hip ratio. It seems that these women saw significant improvement in their weight and health, just because they *thought* they were doing something healthy.

This study shows that the placebo response can be powerful enough to change objective body measurements including weight and levels of body fat.

Can we use this to our advantage? You bet. Here are some simple mental exercises designed to harness the power of the placebo response, and get you in the best frame of mind for fat loss and improved fitness success.

See It

There's an old adage: 'What you resist, persists.' The idea here is that if you tend to focus on the things in your life that you *don't* want, then the very act of focusing on them causes them to perpetuate. One quick way to get around this problem is to change your mental tack. Instead of concentrating on, say, not being overweight, put your energy into being slim. Sounds the same? It's not. Essentially, motivation tends to be stronger if we are moving towards something positive rather than attempting to move away from something negative.

So, instead of getting locked into focusing on those physical attributes that you are not happy with, keep in mind the size and shape of the body you really want to have. If it's a trimmer waist and a more muscular upper body you want, then that's the image to keep in mind as you go through the process of change. If you're looking to be fitter and healthier, then hold that as your ultimate goal.

One thing that can help here is to have real images around you that represent the benefits you're aiming for, such a pictures of you when you were in better shape, or even pictures of others (e.g. athletes, sportspeople) you find inspirational. Have a very clear picture in your mind of how you want the new and improved version of you to look.

Once you have this, it's time to move on to the next stage.

Feel It

Now that you have a positive image of the person you want to be, get excited about it. How would you feel if you were slim and healthy now? Plug into your new vision of yourself with all your senses, just as if you were that person right here, right now. Imagine how you would think and feel as this improved version of you.

Once you can truly see and feel this transformed image of you, it's time to take action.

Be It

The final step to manifesting the changes you desire is to do something about them. Behave in a way that is in accordance with the person you see and feel. As much as possible, act in a manner you would expect this transformed image of you to behave. Eat the health-giving foods the 'new' you eats. Be active and take exercise just as you would if you were already in great shape. Do anything and everything that is representative of the person you aspire to be. Thinking and acting positively regarding your body can be a powerful force for change. However, we can also apply this principle to external factors, too, including the food we eat and the activities we engage in.

MAKE FRIENDS WITH FOOD

One of the secrets to using your brain as a force for good is to keep a positive mental attitude. Applying this principle to our diet can be important, because many of the messages we get from health professionals regarding diet are essentially negative. A great deal of dietary advice meted out by doctors and dieticians is centred around telling us what *not* to do. Even in this book, for instance, I've warned you off all sorts of foods including refined sugar, starchy foods, margarine, trans fats, MSG and artificial sweeteners.

However, we don't need to dwell on those foodstuffs. Rather than focusing on what *not* to eat, I suggest concentrating on what *to* eat. As already mentioned, concentrating on doing something, rather than on *not* doing something, is a powerful motivator for action. Remember that, while food may have been the undoing of you, it can also be your salvation. It's a question of making the right food choices. Now you are in no doubt about which foods are most likely to allow you to achieve your goals, it's important to see these foods as your allies in the quest to shed fat and enhance your health.

EATING MINDFULLY

Another mental approach that can reap dividends in terms of accelerated fat loss is 'mindful eating'. Some of us eat in quite an unconscious or 'mindless' way, which may be more habit-driven than provoked by true hunger or our nutritional needs. Some of us, for example, may eat as a result of boredom or stress. Our food choices may also be dictated more by what happens to be in our vicinity, rather than what we know is good for us. Eating mindfully helps us fulfil our nutritional needs quite appropriately, and has been found to be associated with improved weight control over time.[2]

Here are some tips on how to eat mindfully:

- Before you eat a meal or snack, stop for a moment to ask yourself if there is genuine hunger there, or if something else is driving your eating, such as boredom or habit.
- At home, serve food on smallish plates, and focus on the quality of the food you are eating, not its quantity.
- When eating, stay focused on the food as much as possible, avoiding external distractions such as work, reading, internet surfing and the TV.
- Eat slowly, chew thoroughly and savour the food you eat (see Chapter 6 for more on this).
- Eat until comfortably full, in the knowledge that if you get genuinely hungry before the next meal, it's

perfectly OK to snack on something healthy such as some nuts.

One unconscious driver of unnecessary eating that is worth looking out for and neutralising is the notion that we need to finish everything on our plate. A common cause of this can be the messages we may have received in childhood about the importance of not wasting food, particularly in light of the plight of starving children somewhere in the third world. I in no way wish to make light of this issue, but the fact remains that eating more than you need to in no way helps starving children (or anyone else) somewhere else. Being mindful of the fact that overeating helps no one (save food manufacturers and retailers) can be all that it takes to rid yourself of your 'clear the plate' mentality.

EMBRACE EXERCISE

Some of us may have grown up in an environment where exercise was used as a punishment. Or maybe some sporting failures as a child caused us to form the belief that activity and exercise were 'not for us'. If you have any of these mental barriers to exercise, it's important to remind yourself that the rules have changed.

Whatever your past experiences, you can still delight in the fact that a 20- to 30-minute walk at lunchtime in your work clothes is likely to be doing you the power of good. The 12-minute regime advocated in the previous chapter need not strike fear in your heart, either. In fact, you may find yourself focusing on the fact that as the weeks pass you're making real and discernable progress in what you are able to achieve in those dozen minutes. Not to mention the positive effects this relatively brief workout is having on how you look with your clothes off.

THINK YOURSELF FIT?

The chambermaid experiment discussed above suggests that it's possible to think ourselves slim. Is it possible to think ourselves fit, too? One approach which has shown distinct promise here is *visualisation*. Some sportspeople (e.g. golfers) use visualisation to mentally rehearse shots in an effort to improve technique and performance. There is some evidence that visualisation has the potential to improve muscular strength, too.

In one study, individuals underwent training of the 'abductor' muscles in their little finger.[3] These muscles move the little finger away from the other fingers. Another group underwent no physical training, but performed 'mental abduction' of the little finger. In other words, they imagined that they were sticking out their little finger, without actually doing it.

At the end of the 12-week study, the group who underwent physical training of their little finger saw a 53 per cent increase in the strength of this movement. The group who only imagined the movement, however, saw a 35 per cent increase in strength. This study also employed a group who mentally trained their biceps muscle. Strength increased here, too, though to a lesser degree (13.5 per cent).

In another study of similar design, training of the little finger abductor muscles increased the strength of this movement by 30 per cent.[4] Imagining the movement led to a 22 per cent increase in strength. Both real training and imagined training led to an increase in strength in the little finger on the other (untrained) side of the body, too.

In another piece of research, visualisation outperformed actual physical training in terms of strengthening the muscles that move the ankle.[5]

What are we to learn from this? Well, just imagining performing exercise appears to have some ability to enhance strength. Even if the effect is small, getting stronger without doing any physical work is an attractive proposition. How might you apply this?

Imagine you're sitting on a train or lying in the sun doing not very much at all. Close your eyes and imagine yourself going through the 12-minute exercise regime outlined in the preceding chapter. Or choose some other exercise or activity you particularly enjoy. Make it as real as possible. Imagine yourself in the real setting wearing appropriate clothing. As you perform the exercise or activity in your mind's eye, see and feel your muscles moving and contracting as you go through each of the exercises. Aim to practise this at least once a day, but don't stop there if you feel inclined to do it more often.

KEEP A DIARY

One quick habit that can help you maintain healthy habits is to keep a diary. Each day, jot down in a notebook, smart-phone or computer what you've eaten and drunk over the course of that day, and the activity you have taken. This simple act can help you feel more accountable for your actions, making it less likely that you're going to fall off the wagon.

You might also add notes about the positive changes you have experienced, both in terms of fat loss (however you choose to assess this) and other factors that may be important to you such as greater energy, enhanced productivity, better sleep and enhanced strength and physical performance during exercise. Reviewing your diary from time to time can help to remind you of the benefits you're experiencing, which can also help maintain the healthy behaviours that have brought those benefits about.

DIET IS A FOUR-LETTER WORD

The information contained in this book is a scientifically based route-map to permanent fat loss and improved wellbeing. The principles here have been successfully tested on the ground with countless men. The principles work, but obviously only if you apply them – *consistently*.

We know that diets don't work, so my strong advice to you is not to see *Waist Disposal* as a diet. The word 'diet' can, for some people, conjure up images of some strict and unsustainable regime. For this reason I encourage you to see the suggestions here not as some stringent, restrictive regime that will inevitably come to an end in a few weeks or months, but a healthy way of eating to be used for lifelong benefit.

At the same time, I know that most of us don't like the thought of committing to change until we know it's something that we're actually going to want to sustain. So, with this in mind, I suggest you resolve, in the first instance, to give the information and advice here a trial of 30 days. This will be long enough for you to judge the benefits to be had from applying the advice. How you judge the progress you've made is up to you, but examples include:

- **the amount of weight you have lost**

- **the change in your waist size**

- **the extent of your fat loss as adjudged by skin-fold thickness measurements (see Chapter 1)**

- **the increase in the number of press-ups/sit-ups you can do in a minute**

- **the satisfaction you get from seeing the distinct change in the look of your body clothed and naked**

- **a feeling of enhanced energy and wellbeing.**

In all likelihood, reflecting on the benefits you have gained make incorporating these changes an attractive proposition in the long term. Even so, my experience tells me that there are some common banana skins that can trip us up. We're going to go through the most common ones, and how to counter them.

HUNGER

I can't tell you how important it is not to allow yourself to get too hungry if you want to eat healthily. It's because I think it's so important that I've mentioned it several times in this book already. For example, in the second chapter (The Calorie Trap) I cited hunger as a major reason why diets fail. I've warned against getting too hungry before your lunch or evening meal. I've devoted a whole chapter to how to ensure that rampant hunger never gets the opportunity to bite (Chapter 6).

If there's a belief still inside you that equates hunger with weight loss, then this belief needs expunging from your psyche *now*.

The reality is that *not being very hungry* is a key to successful fat loss – it's what allows individuals to eat appropriate amounts of the right foods. Eating truly healthy foods frequently enough (as covered in Chapter 6) is essential if you are to enjoy the permanent benefits *Waist Disposal* promises.

THERE'S NO REASON TO BE RIGID

Initially, I suggest quite a strict approach to this regime. The results will be better that way, and it can help to stabilise blood-sugar levels (and therefore combat false hunger) more quickly. But imagine now you're six weeks into your new life and have lost 6 kg, a couple of inches off your waist, and are already seeing your torso and arms have a much more defined look about them. Does that mean you absolutely have to eschew the sandwich-based working lunch on Wednesday, or go without a glass or two of red wine with your dinner on Friday night? Of course not.

There's no need to let these sorts of things derail you. In the long term, remember that it's what you eat *most of the time*, not some of it, that will determine your body composition and health. The important thing here is that you do not let these incidents cloud the bigger picture. Rather than focusing on individual meals or the odd drinking session, keep an overview of the totality of your diet. See whatever you eat in the context of your diet as a whole. Aim, in the long term, to ensure that at least 80 per cent of your food and drink comes from items in the 'consume freely' categories such as meat, fish, eggs, green vegetables, nuts, berries, water and naturally decaffeinated tea and coffee.

WHY THE ODD SPLURGE WILL NOT NECESSARILY MAKE YOU FATTER

A key tenet of *Waist Disposal* is that weight loss is not the goal, but fat loss is. Just as when weight is lost it won't necessarily be fat (particularly in the initial stages of weight loss), when weight goes up, that won't necessarily be fat, either. On a low-carb regime, some initial weight loss will come from depletion in the stores of glycogen (a form of starch), a storage fuel found mainly in the liver and muscles. When carb intake is cut, the body will tend to mobilise glycogen, effectively lowering glycogen stores and weight as it does so.

Now, imagine you have been eating a relatively low-carb diet for a while, and now have relatively low glycogen stores. And let's say one night you decide to treat yourself to a pasta supper and some beers. What all the carb will do, basically, is help refill your glycogen stores. Only if you continue eating lots of carb are you likely to then start converting it to fat. So, after a bit of a carb-fest, you may well be a bit heavier in the morning, but it's unlikely you're going to be any *fatter*. Also, when the body stores glycogen, it stores fluid with it – something which can also cause weight to bounce up a touch.

Some individuals keen on keeping a track of their weight can be horrified when they find that their weight has increased by, say, a couple of pounds from one day to the next. This can't be due to fat accumulation, though. A pound of fat contains 3,500 calories. So, in theory, to add two pounds of fat the calorific excess would be 7,000 calories. In the space of a day, that would be a stretch even for someone purposefully gorging themselves on the unhealthiest foods they could find. In reality, when weight springs up like this, it's likely to be down to the body storing a little more glycogen as well as the fluid that goes with it.

THE PROBLEM WITH PROPAGANDA

Another major reason for dietary default concerns what I regard as nutritional propaganda – basically, erroneous dietary advice and information, some of which comes from organisations that may be more motivated by profit than solving your personal health concerns. The nutritional principles espoused in this book often run counter to conventional nutritional 'wisdom'. The chances are that, soon after putting this book down, you will, for instance, read or hear something that alerts you, yet again, to the perils of eating animal fat, while at the same time exalting quite suspect foods such as wholemeal bread, low-fat milk, processed breakfast cereals with added sugar and salt, margarine and artificial sweeteners. That's business.

I know from my experience in practice how powerful and pervasive these erroneous messages can be. That is why I have done my best in this book to set the nutritional record straight through a thorough appraisal of the science. Even armed with this information, it can sometimes take a strong person and quite a degree of conviction to reject, for instance, the doctor's or dietician's recommendation to eschew red meat and butter because of an 'elevated' cholesterol level. I don't encourage you to reject what health professionals say out of hand. However, I do suggest a degree of healthy scepticism.

I am a great believer in individuals being their own advocates. Knowledge is power, as they say, and that is partly why this book takes a frank, science-based approach. The hundreds of research studies referred to in *Waist Disposal* are included, at least in part, to give you the confidence that the strategies presented here are effective and safe. But, as I mentioned back in the introduction to this book, it can sometimes be a stretch to remember the scientific detail that underpins the advice given here. It was also in the introduction that I made the point that, leaving the science aside for a moment, logic dictates that the best diet for us will be one based on the foods we have been eating longest in terms of our time on this planet. You can be confident in the fact that the recommendations here are not just supported by science, but common sense, too. Apply the advice here and you can look forward to seeing the benefits in the form of a leaner, stronger, altogether healthier body.

KEEPING THE 'PRIMAL PICTURE' IN MIND

Throughout this book evidence has been presented which demonstrates that the healthiest diet is one which mirrors our ancient, evolutionary diet. It can sometimes be helpful to use a mental picture to remind us, from time to time, of what sort of a diet that was. Just conjure up now a picture of our early ancestors, perhaps sitting around a fire, feasting on some primal fare. What can you see? Meat? Maybe fish? How about some fruit, vegetable matter and nuts? Such visions will be utterly plausible for most of us.

What you *won't* be able to see, though, is our distant relatives tucking into sandwiches, bagels, biscuits, bowls of breakfast cereal or platefuls of pasta, all washed down with soft drinks or cappuccinos. Having this image in your mind will help you to make rapid, accurate choices about the very best foods to eat, not just now, but for the rest of your life. Looking to our nutritional past is key to ensuring a vibrantly healthy present and future.

BACK TO BASICS

- Having a positive mental attitude can have real, discernable benefits for the body in terms of health and weight.

- Visualising and feeling the positive changes you desire, and acting in accordance with them, can accelerate your progress.

- Viewing food and exercise in a positive light, and eating mindfully, can also help the process of change.

- Do not concern yourself with occasional slip-ups and indulgences: it's what you eat most of the time that's important.

- In the long term, aim to base 80 per cent of your diet on 'freely permitted' foodstuffs.

- Keeping in mind the diet of our evolutionary ancestors will help you make accurate and quick decisions about appropriate foods, and help you in your quest to transform your body into something lean, strong and vibrantly healthy.

WAIST DISPOSAL AT A GLANCE

There's a lot of information in this book, and sometimes focusing on the essentials can help us to 'stick with the programme', and achieve lasting success in terms of fat loss, enhanced fitness and body composition and other benefits. To this end, here is the whole of *Waist Disposal* condensed into 11 key principles.

You might want to copy these central tenets and put them in a prominent place, like on your desk or fridge door. Or perhaps transcribe them into a notebook, PDA or smart-phone for easy reference.

1. **Body weight and the body mass index do not reflect body *composition*, and are therefore limited in their usefulness. Estimations of *body fatness* and *waist circumference* are much more relevant measurements in terms of assessing health and fat-loss progress.**

2. **Whether a food is fattening or not depends not just on the calories it contains, but on the *form* those calories take, as well as how good the food is at *sating the appetite*. Forget about counting calories, and concentrate instead on eating a diet rich in foods that counter the accumulation of fat in the body, and at the same time quell the appetite most effectively.**

3. **The *chief fat-storage hormone* in the body is *insulin*, which is secreted most plentifully in response to *carbohydrate* (sugars and starches). The most fattening foods are therefore those that cause most disruption to blood-sugar and insulin levels. These include foods with added sugar, as well as starchy foods such as bread, potato, rice, pasta, noodles, crackers and breakfast cereals. Eat as little of these foods as possible.**

4. *Fat is not inherently fattening,* and certain fats (e.g. omega-3 fats) have distinct health benefits. Fats to avoid include refined vegetable oils (in excess) and industrially-produced processed fats such as 'trans' fat (in any amount). Otherwise, eat fat freely.

5. *Protein has superior appetite-sating properties* to carbohydrate, and causes *less insulin* secretion too. As such, a protein-rich diet can therefore assist *fat loss.* Protein is also essential for the maintenance and growth of muscle tissue, which is important for improved body composition. Protein (e.g. meat, fish and eggs) should be eaten freely.

6. *Vegetables* (other than the potato) are, on the whole, *nutritious foods that tend not to cause much disruption to sugar and insulin.* They, generally speaking, should be eaten freely.

7. Eat enough (in terms of volume) and frequently enough to *satisfy your appetite fully.* In particular, ensure that you do not let your appetite run out of control. This may require healthy snacking (e.g. nuts) between meals, especially between lunch and dinner. At the same time, ensure you eat only when you are truly hungry (not when bored or in need of distraction). *Eat 'mindfully'* – focus on what you eat, savour food, and chew it thoroughly.

8. *Make water your prime fluid,* and keep a supply of this close to you (e.g. a bottle of water on your desk). Coffee, tea and herb/fruit teas are generally healthy options too.

9. Incorporate *brisk walking* into your daily schedule as much as possible, even in short bursts. In addition, engage in *resistance exercise* (such as the *12-minute exercise routine* outlined in chapter 10) regularly.

10. Adopt a *positive mental attitude* regarding the changes that you're making, and maintain a *positive image* and sense *of the transformation you're seeking* to achieve.

11. Keep in mind that the most healthy behaviours are generally those that are in accordance with our evolutionary past – so *live and eat as 'primally' as possible!*

REFERENCES

CHAPTER 1

1. Flegal, K M *et al.*, 'Cause-Specific Excess Deaths Associated With Underweight, Overweight, and Obesity', *JAMA* 2007; 298(17): 2028–37

2. Orpana, H M *et al.*, 'BMI and Mortality: Results from a National Longitudinal Study of Canadian Adults', *Obesity* 18 June 2009 [Epub ahead of print publication]

3. Troiano, R P *et al.*, 'The relationship between body weight and mortality: a quantitative analysis of combined information from existing studies', *Int J Obes Relat Metab Disord* 1996; 20: 63–75

4. Pischon, T *et al.*, 'General and abdominal adiposity and risk of death in Europe', *N Engl J Med* 2008; 358(20): 2105-20

5. Canoy, D, 'Distribution of body fat and risk of coronary heart disease in men and women', *Curr Opin Cardiol* 2008; 23(6): 591–98

6. Pischon, T *et al.*, op cit

7. Whitmer, R A *et al.*, 'Central obesity and increased risk of dementia more than three decades later', *Neurology* 2008; 71(14): 1057–64

8. Fisman, E Z and A Tenenbaum (eds), 'Impaired glucose metabolism and cerebrovascular diseases', in *Cardiovascular Diabetology, Metabolic and Inflammatory Facets, Advances in Cardiology*, Karger. 2008; 45: 107–113

CHAPTER 2

1. Young, C M *et al.*, 'Effect of body composition and other parameters in obese young men of carbohydrate level

of reduction diet', *Am J Clin Nutr* 1971; 24: 290–96

2. Lean, M E *et al.*, 'Weight loss with high and low carbohydrate 1200 kcal diets in free living women', *Eur J Clin Nutr* 1997; 51: 243–48

3. Wien, M A *et al.*, 'Almonds vs complex carbohydrates in a weight reduction program', *Int J Obes* 2003; 27: 1365–72

4. Kennedy, A R, *et al.*, 'A high-fat, ketogenic diet induces a unique metabolic state in mice', *Am J Physiol Endocrinol Metab* 2007; 292: E1724–E1739

5. Redman, L M *et al.*, 'Metabolic and behavioral compensations in response to caloric restriction: implications for the maintenance of weight loss', *PLoS One* 2009; 4(2): e4377

6. Weyer C *et al.*, 'Energy metabolism after two years of energy restriction: the biosphere 2 experiment', *Am J Clin Nutr* 2000; 72(4): 946–53

7. Redman, L M *et al.*, op cit; Weyer, C *et al.*, op cit.

CHAPTER 3

1. Wannamethee, S G *et al.*, 'Modifiable lifestyle factors and the metabolic syndrome in older men: effects of lifestyle changes', *Journal of the American Geriatrics Society* 2006; 54(12): 1909–14

2. Kechagias, S *et al.*, 'Fast-food-based hyper-alimentation can induce rapid and profound elevation of serum alanine aminotranferase in healthy subjects', *Gut* 2008; 57(5): 649–54

3. Scribner, K B *et al.*, 'Long-term effects of dietary glycemic index on adiposity, energy metabolism and physical activity in mice', *Am J Physiol Endocrinol Metab* 2008; 295(5): E1126–31

4. Roberts, S B, 'High-glycemic index foods, hunger, and obesity: is there a connection?', *Nutrition Review* 2000;

58: 163–69

5. Westman, E *et al.*, 'Low carbohydrate nutrition and metabolism', *Am J Clin Nutr* 2007; 86: 276–84

6. Sondike, S B *et al.*, 'Effects of a low-carbohydrate diet on weight loss and cardiovascular risk factor in overweight adolescents', *J Pediatr* 2003; 142(3): 253–58

7. Brehm, B J *et al.*, 'A randomized trial comparing a very low carbohydrate diet and a calorie-restricted low fat diet on body weight and cardiovascular risk factors in healthy women', *J Clin Endocrinol Metab* 2003; 88: 1617–23

8. Foster, G D *et al.*, 'A randomized trial of a low-carbohydrate diet for obesity', *N Engl J Med* 2003; 348: 2082–90

9. Yancy, W S Jr *et al.*, 'A low carbohydrate, ketogenic diet versus a low-fat diet to treat obesity and hyperlipidemia. A randomized, controlled trial', *Ann Intern Med* 2004; 140: 69–77

10. Stern, L *et al.*, 'The effects of low-carbohydrate versus conventional weight-loss diets in severely obese adults: one-year follow-up of a randomized trial', *Ann Intern Med* 2004; 140: 778–85

11. Gardner, C D *et al.*, 'Comparison of the Atkins, Zone, Ornish, and LEARN Diets for Change in Weight and Related Risk Factors Among Overweight Pre-menopausal Women: The A TO Z Weight Loss Study: A Randomized Trial', *JAMA* 2007; 297: 969–77

12. Shai, I *et al.*, 'Weight Loss with a Low-Carbohydrate, Mediterranean, or Low-Fat Diet', *N Engl J Med* 2008; 359: 229–41

13. Foster, G D, Stern, L and Shai, I, op cit

14. Foster, G D and Stern, L, op cit

15. Stern, L, op cit

16. Foster, G D, op cit

17. Yancy, W S and Gardner, C D, op cit
18. Bravata, D M *et al.*, 'Efficacy and safety of low-carbohydrate diets: a systematic review', *JAMA* 2003; 289(14): 1837–50
19. Krieger, J W *et al.*, 'Effects of variation in protein and carbohydrate intake on body mass and composition during energy restriction: a meta-regression', *Am J Clin Nutr* 2006; 83(2): 260–74
20. Brand-Miller, J *et al.*, 'The Glycemic Index and Cardiovascular Disease Risk', *Current Atherosclerosis Reports* 2007; 9: 479–85
21. Mente, A *et al.*, 'A Systematic Review of the Evidence Supporting a Causal Link Between Dietary Factors and Coronary Heart Disease', *Arch Intern Med* 2009; 169(7): 659–69
22. Grieb, P *et al.*, 'Long-term consumption of a carbohydrate-restricted diet does not induce deleterious metabolic effects', *Nutr Res* 2008; 28(12): 825–33
23. Halton, T L *et al.*, 'Low-carbohydrate-diet score and risk of type 2 diabetes in women', *Am J Clin Nutr* 2008; 87: 339–46
24. Krishnan, S *et al.*, 'Glycemic Index, Glycemic Load, and Cereal Fiber Intake and Risk of Type 2 Diabetes in US Black Women', *Arch Intern Med* 2007; 167(21): 2304–09
25. Barclay, A W *et al.*, 'Glycemic index, glycemic load, and chronic disease risk – a meta-analysis of observational studies', *Am J Clin Nutr* 2008; 87(3): 627–37
26. Wu, W *et al.*, 'The brain in the age of the old: The hippocampal formation is targeted differentially by diseases of late life', *Ann Neurol* 2008; 64: 698–706
27. Whitmer, R A *et al.*, 'Central obesity and increased risk of dementia more than three decades later', *Neurology*

2008; 71(14): 1057–64

28. National Diet and Nutrition Survey. UK Office of National Statistics, 2004

29. Cordain, L *et al.*, 'Plant-animal subsistence ratios and macronutrient energy estimations in worldwide hunter-gatherer diets', *Am J Clin Nutr* 2000; 71(3): 682–92

30. Drewnowski, A, 'Concept of a nutritious food: toward a nutrient density score', *Am J Clin Nutr* 2005; 82: 721–32

CHAPTER 4

1. Melanson, K J *et al.*, 'Blood glucose patterns and appetite in time-blinded humans: carbohydrate versus fat', *Am J Physiol* 1999; 277(2 Pt 2): R337–45

2. Cecil J E *et al.*, 'Comparison of the effects of a high-fat and high-carbohydrate soup delivered orally and intragastrically on gastric emptying, appetite, and eating behaviour', *Physiol Behav* 1999; 67(2): 299–306

3. Sabaté, J, 'Nut consumption and body weight', *Am J Clin Nutr* 2003; 78(3 Suppl): 647S–650S

4. Wien, M A *et al.*, 'Almonds vs complex carbohydrates in a weight reduction program', *Int J Obes* 2003; 27: 1365–72

5. Pirozzo, S *et al.*, 'Advice on low-fat diets for obesity', *Cochrane Database Syst Rev* 2002; (2): CD003640

6. Willett, C *et al.*, 'Dietary fat is not a major determinant of body fat', *Am J Med* 2002; 113(9B): 47S–59S

7. Keys, A, 'Coronary heart disease in seven countries', *Circulation* 1970; 41(suppl. 1): 1–211

8. Paul, O *et al.*, 'A longitudinal study of coronary heart disease', *Circulation* 1963; 28: 20–31

9. Gordon, T, 'The Framingham Diet Study: diet and the regulation of serum cholesterol', in *The Framingham Study: An Epidemiological Investigation*

of *Cardiovascular Disease*, Section 24. US Government Printing Office, Washington, DC, 1970

10. Medalie, J H *et al.*, 'Five-year myocardial infarction incidence. II. Association of single variables to age and birthplace', *Journal of Chronic Diseases* 1973; 26(6): 325–49

11. Morris, I N *et al.*, 'Diet and heart: a postscript', *BMJ* 1977; 2: 1307–14

12. Yano, K *et al.*, 'Dietary intake and the risk of coronary heart disease in Japanese men living in Hawaii', *Am J Clin Nutr* 1978; 31: 1270–79

13. Garcia-Palmieri, M R *et al.*, 'Relationship of dietary intake to subsequent coronary heart disease incidence: The Puerto Rico Heart Health Program', *Am J Clin Nutr* 1980; 33(8): 1818–27

14. Gordon, T *et al.*, 'Diet and its relation to coronary heart disease in three populations', *Circulation* 1981; 63; 500–15

15. Shekelle, R B *et al.*, 'Diet, serum cholesterol, and death from coronary heart disease: the Western Electric Study', *N Engl J Med* 1981; 304: 65–70

16. McGee, D L *et al.*, 'Ten-year incidence of coronary heart disease in the Honolulu Heart Program: relationship to nutrient intake', *American Journal of Epidemiology* 1984; 119: 667–76

17. Kromhout, D *et al.*, 'Diet, prevalence and 10-year mortality from coronary heart disease in 871 middle-aged men: the Zutphen Study', *American Journal of Epidemiology* 1984; 119: 733–741

18. Kushi, L H *et al.*, 'Diet and 20-year mortality from coronary heart disease: the Ireland-Boston Diet-Heart Study', *N Engl J Med* 1985; 312: 811–18

19. Lapidus, L *et al.*, 'Dietary habits in relation to incidence of cardiovascular disease and death in women: a 12-

year follow-up of participants in the population study of women in Gothenburg, Sweden', *Am J Clin Nutr* 1986; 44(4): 444–48

20. Khaw, K T *et al.*, 'Dietary fiber and reduced ischemic heart disease mortality rates in men and women: a 12-year prospective study', *American Journal of Epidemiology* 1987; 126(6): 1093–1102

21. Farchi, G *et al.*, 'Diet and 20-year mortality in two rural population groups of middle-aged men in Italy', *Am J Clin Nutr* 1989; 50(5): 1095–1103

22. Posner, B M *et al.*, 'Dietary lipid predictors of coronary heart disease in men: the Framingham Study', *Arch Intern Med* 1991; 151: 1181–87

23. Dolecek, T A, 'Epidemiological evidence of relationships between dietary polyunsaturated fatty acids and mortality in the multiple risk factor intervention trial', *Proceedings of the Society for Experimental Biology and Medicine* 1992; 200(2): 177–82

24. Fehily, A M *et al.*, 'Diet and incident ischaemic heart disease: the Caerphilly Study', *British Journal of Nutrition* 1993; 69: 303–314

25. Goldbourt, U *et al.*, 'Factors predictive of long-term coronary heart disease mortality among 10,059 male Israeli civil servants and municipal employees: a 23-year mortality follow-up in the Israeli Ischemic Heart Disease Study', *Cardiology* 1993; 82: 100–21

26. Esrey, K L *et al.*, 'Relationship between dietary intake and coronary heart disease mortality: Lipid Research Clinics Prevalence Follow-Up Study', *Journal of Clinical Epidemiology* 1996; 49(2): 211–16

27. Ascherio, A *et al.*, 'Dietary fat and risk of coronary heart disease in men: cohort follow-up study in the United States', *BMJ* 1996; 313: 84–90

28. Pietinen, P *et al.*, 'Intake of fatty acids and risk of

coronary heart disease in a cohort of Finnish men: the Aipha-Tocopherol, Beta-Carotene Cancer Prevention Study', *American Journal of Epidemiology* 1997; 145: 876–87

29. Hu, F B *et al.*, 'Dietary fat intake and the risk of coronary heart disease in women', *N Eng J Med* 1997; 337(21): 1491–99
30. Tanasescu, M *et al.*, 'Dietary fat and cholesterol and the risk of cardiovascular disease among women with type 2 diabetes', *Am J Clin Nutr* 2004; 79: 999–1005
31. Laaksonen, D E *et al.*, 'Prediction of cardiovascular mortality in middle-aged men by dietary and serum linoleic and polyunsaturated fatty acids', *Arch of Intern Med* 2005; 165: 193–99
32. Tucker, K L *et al.*, 'The Combination of High Fruit and Vegetable and Low Saturated Fat Intakes Is More Protective against Mortality in Aging Men than Is Either Alone: The Baltimore Longitudinal Study of Aging', *J Nutr* 2005; 135: 556–61
33. Leosdottir, M *et al.*, 'Dietary fat intake and early mortality patterns – data from The Malmo Diet and Cancer Study', *Journal of Internal Medicine* 2005; 258: 153–65
34. McGee, D L, Kushi, L H, Esrey, K L, Tucker, K L, op cit
35. Mozaffarian, D *et al.*, 'Dietary fats, carbohydrate, and progression of coronary atherosclerosis in postmenopausal women', *Am J Clin Nutr* 2004; 80(5): 1175–84
36. Morrison, L M, 'A nutritional program for prolongation of life in coronary atherosclerosis', *JAMA* 1955; 159(15): 1425–28
37. Ball, K P *et al.*, 'Low-fat diet in myocardial infarction: a controlled trial', *Lancet* 1965; 2: 501–504
38. Hood, B *et al.*, 'Long-term prognosis in essential

hypercholesterolemia: the effect of strict diet', *Acta Medica Scandanavica* 1965; 178 (2): 161–73

39. Rose, G A, *et al.*, 'Corn oil in treatment of ischaemic heart disease', *BMJ* 1965; 1: 1531–33

40. Christakis, G *et al.*, 'Effect of the Anti-Coronary Club on coronary heart disease risk factor status', *JAMA* 1966; 198(6): 597–604

41. Bierenbaum, M L *et al.*, 'Modified fat dietary management of the young male with coronary disease. A five year-report', *JAMA* 1967; 202(13): 1119–23

42. National Diet Heart Study. Final report. *Circulation* 1968; 37(3 Suppl): 1–428

43. 'Controlled trial of soya-bean oil in myocardial infarction', *Lancet* 1968; 2(7570): 693–99

44. Dayton, S *et al.*, 'A controlled clinical trial of a diet high in unsaturated fat in preventing complications of atherosclerosis', *Circulation* 1969; 40 (Suppl. II): 1–63

45. Leren, P, 'The Oslo Diet-Heart Study: Eleven Year Report', *Circulation* 1970; 42: 935–42

46. Miettinen, M *et al.*, 'Effect of cholesterol-lowering diet on mortality from coronary heart disease and other causes. A twelve-year clinical trial in men and women', *Lancet* 1972; 2(7782): 835–38

47. Woodhill, J M *et al.*, 'Low fat, low cholesterol diet in secondary prevention of coronary heart disease', *Advances in Experimental Medicine and Biology* 1978; 109: 317–30

48. Turpenien, O *et al.*, 'Dietary prevention of coronary heart disease: the Finnish Mental Hospital Study', *Int J Epidemiol* 1979: 8: 9–118

49. Hjermann, I *et al.*, 'Effect of diet and smoking in the incidence of coronary heart disease', *Lancet* 1981: ii: 1303–10

50. World Health Organization European Collaborative

Group, European collaborative trial of multifactorial prevention of coronary heart disease. *Lancet* 1986: 1: 869–72

51. Frantz, I D Jr *et al.*, 'Test of effect of lipid lowering by diet on cardiovascular risk. The Minnesota coronary survey', *Arteriosclerosis* 1989; 9: 129–35

52. Burr, M L *et al.*, 'Effects of changes in fat, fish, and fibre intakes on death and myocardial reinfarction: diet and reinfarction trial (DART)', *Lancet* 1989; 2(8666): 757–61

53. Strandberg, T E *et al.*, 'Long-term mortality after 5-year multifactorial primary prevention of cardiovascular diseases in middle-aged men', *JAMA* 1991: 266: 1225–29

54. Watts, G F *et al.*, 'Effects on coronary artery disease of lipid-lowering diet, or diet plus cholestyramine, in the St Thomas' atherosclerosis regression study (STARS)', *Lancet* 1992; 339(8793): 563–69

55. Neaton, J D, Blackburn, H, Jacobs, D *et al.*, 'Serum cholesterol level and mortality: findings for men screened in the Multiple Risk Factor Intervention Trial', *Arch Intern Med* 1992: 152: 1490–1500

56. De Lorgeril, M *et al.*, 'Mediterranean alpha-linolenic acid-rich diet in secondary prevention of coronary heart disease', *Lancet* 1994; 343(8911): 1454–59

57. Howard, B V *et al.*, 'Low-Fat Dietary Pattern and Risk of Cardiovascular Disease: The Women's Health Initiative Randomized Controlled Dietary Modification Trial', *JAMA* 2006; 295: 655–66

58. Mozaffarian, D, Ball, K P, Dayton, S, Woodhill, J M, Strandberg, T E and Neaton J D *et al.*, op cit

59. Hooper, L *et al.*, 'Dietary intake and prevention of cardiovascular disease: systematic review', *BMJ* 2001; 322(7289): 757–630

60. Mente, A *et al.*, 'A Systematic Review of the Evidence Supporting a Causal Link Between Dietary Factors and Coronary Heart Disease', *Arch Intern Med* 2009; 169(7): 659–69

61. Scientific steering committee on behalf of the Simon Broome Register group, 'Risk of fatal coronary heart disease in familial hypercholesterolaemia', *BMJ* 1991; 303: 893–96

62. Forette, F *et al.*, 'The prognostic significance of isolated systolic hypertension in the elderly. Results of a ten-year longitudinal survey', *Clinical and Experimental Hypertension. Part A, Theory and Practice* 1982; 4: 1177–91

63. Siegel, D *et al.*, 'Predictors of cardiovascular events and mortality in the Systolic Hypertension in the Elderly Program pilot project', *American Journal of Epidemiology* 1987; 126: 385–89

64. Nissinen, A *et al.*, 'Risk factors for cardiovascular disease among 55 to 74 year-old Finnish men: a 10-year follow-up', *Annals of Medicine* 1989; 21: 239–40

65. Krumholz, H M *et al.*, 'Lack of association between cholesterol and coronary heart disease mortality and morbidity and all-cause mortality in persons older than 70 years', *JAMA* 1994; 272: 1335–40

66. Weijenberg, M P *et al.*, 'Serum total cholesterol and systolic blood pressure as risk factors for mortality from ischemic heart disease among elderly men and women', *Journal of Clinical Epidemiology* 1994; 47: 197–205

67. Simons, L A *et al.*, 'Diabetes, mortality and coronary heart disease in the prospective Dubbo study of Australian elderly', *Australian and New Zealand Journal of Medicine* 1996; 26: 66–74

68. Weijenberg, M P *et al.*, 'Total and high density lipoprotein

cholesterol as risk factors for coronary heart disease in elderly men during 5 years of follow-up. The Zutphen Elderly Study', *American Journal of Epidemiology* 1996; 143: 151-58

69. Simons, L A *et al.*, 'Cholesterol and other lipids predict coronary heart disease and ischaemic stroke in the elderly, but only in those below 70 years', *Atherosclerosis* 2001; 159: 201-208

70. Abbott, R D *et al.*, 'Age-related changes in risk factor effects on the incidence of coronary heart disease', *Annals of Epidemiology* 2002; 12: 173-81

71. Zimetbaum, P *et al.*, 'Plasma lipids and lipoproteins and the incidence of cardiovascular disease in the very elderly. The Bronx aging study', *Arteriosclerosis Thrombosis and Vascular Biology* 1992; 12: 416-23

72. Fried, L P *et al.*, 'Risk factors for 5-year mortality in older adults: the Cardiovascular Health Study', *JAMA* 1998; 279: 585-92

73. Chyou, P H *et al.*, 'Serum cholesterol concentrations and all-cause mortality in older people', *Age and Ageing* 2000; 29: 69-74

74. Menotti, A *et al.*, 'Cardiovascular risk factors and 10-year all-cause mortality in elderly European male populations; the FINE study', *European Heart Journal* 2001; 22: 573-79

75. Räihä, I *et al.*, 'Effect of serum lipids, lipoproteins, and apolipoproteins on vascular and nonvascular mortality in the elderly', *Arteriosclerosis Thrombosis and Vascular Biology* 1997; 17: 1224-32

76. Brescianini, S *et al.*, 'Low total cholesterol and increased risk of dying: are low levels clinical warning signs in the elderly? Results from the Italian Longitudinal Study on Aging', *Journal of the American Geriatrics Society* 2003; 51(7): 991-96

77. Forette, B *et al.*, 'Cholesterol as risk factor for mortality in elderly women', *Lancet* 1989; 1: 868–70

78. Jonsson, A *et al.*, 'Total cholesterol and mortality after age 80 years', *Lancet* 1997; 350: 1778–79

79. Weverling-Rijnsburger, A W *et al.*, 'Total cholesterol and risk of mortality in the oldest old', *Lancet* 1997; 350: 1119–23

80. Yang, X *et al.*, 'Independent associations between low-density lipoprotein cholesterol and cancer among patients with type 2 diabetes mellitus', *Canadian Medical Association Journal* 2008; 179(5): 427–37

81. Studer, M *et al.*, 'Effect of different antilipidemic agents and diets on mortality', *Arch Intern Med* 2005; 165: 725–30

82. Gillman, M W *et al.*, 'Margarine intake and subsequent coronary heart disease in men', *Epidemiology* 1997; 8(2): 144–49

83. Willett, W C *et al.*, 'Intake of trans fatty acids and risk of coronary heart disease among women', *Lancet* 1993; 341(8845): 581–85

84. Wang, C *et al.*, 'n-3 fatty acids from fish or fish-oil supplements, but not α-linolenic acid, benefit cardiovascular disease outcomes in primary- and secondary-prevention studies: a systematic review', *Am J Clin Nutr* 2006; 84: 5–17

85. Schaefer, E J *et al.*, 'Plasma Phosphatidylcholine Docosahexaenoic Acid Content and Risk of Dementia and Alzheimer Disease: The Framingham Heart Study', *Archives of Neurology* 2006; 63: 1545–50

86. Weber, P C, 'Are we what we eat? Fatty acids in nutrition and in cell membranes: cell functions and disorders induced by dietary conditions', in *Fish fats and your health* (Norway: Svanoy Foundation, 1989): 9–18

87. Raheja, B S *et al.*, 'Significance of the n-6/n-3 ratio for

insulin action in diabetes', *Ann N Y Acad Sci* 1993; 683: 258–71

88. Simopoulos, A P, 'The importance of the ratio of omega-6/omega-3 essential fatty acids', *Biomed Pharmacother* 2002; 56(8): 365–79

89. Cordain, L *et al.*, 'Fatty acid analysis of wild ruminant tissues: evolutionary implications for reducing diet-related chronic disease', *Eur J Clin Nutr* 2002; 56: 181–91

90. Eaton, S B *et al.*, 'Paleolithic nutrition. A consideration of its nature and current implications', *N Engl J Med* 1985; 312: 283–89

91. Simopoulos, A P, Cleland, L G (eds), 'Omega-6/omega-3 Essential Fatty Acid Ratio: The Scientific Evidence', *World Rev Nutr Diet* (Basel); Karger 2003 (vol 92)

92. Guebre-Egziabher, F *et al.*, 'Nutritional intervention to reduce the n-6/n-3 fatty acid ratio increases adiponectin concentration and fatty acid oxidation in healthy subjects', *Eur J Clin Nutr* 2008; 62: 1287–93

93. Kavanagh, K *et al.*, 'Trans fat diet induces insulin resistance in monkeys', Study presented at the Scientific Sessions of the American Diabetes Association in Washington, DC, 2006

94. Pedersen, J I *et al.*, 'Adipose tissue fatty acids and risk of myocardial infarction – a case-control study', *Eur J Clin Nutr* 2000: 54: 618–25

95. Ascherio, A *et al.*, 'Dietary fat and risk of coronary heart disease in men: Cohort follow-up study in the United States', *BMJ* 1996: 313: 84–90

96. Hu, F B *et al.*, 'Dietary fat intake and the risk of coronary heart disease in women', *N Engl J Med* 1997: 337: 1491–99

97. Oomen, C M *et al.*, 'Association between trans fatty acid intake and 10-year risk of coronary heart disease in

the Zutphen Elderly Study: A prospective population-based study', *Lancet* 2001; 357: 746–51

98. Bakker, N *et al.*, 'The Euramic Study Group: Adipose fatty acids and cancers of the breast, prostate and colon: An ecological study', *Cancer* 1997: 72: 587–97

99. Christiansen, E *et al.*, 'Intake of a diet high in trans monounsaturated fatty acids or saturated fatty acids. Effects on postprandial insulinemia and glycemia in obese patients with NIDDM', *Diabetes Care* 1997; 20: 881–87

100.Alstrup, K K *et al.*, 'Differential effects of cis and *trans* fatty acids on insulin release from isolated mouse islets', *Metabolism* 1999: 48: 22–29

101. Salméron, J *et al.*, 'Dietary fat intake and risk of type 2 diabetes in women', *Am J Clin Nutr* 2001; 73: 1019–26

CHAPTER 5

1. Westerterp, K R *et al.*, 'Diet-induced thermogenesis measured over 24 h in a respiration chamber: effect of diet composition', *Int J Obes* 1999; 23: 287–92

2. Hochstenbach-Waelen, A *et al.*, 'Comparison of 2 diets with either 25% or 10% of energy as casein on energy expenditure, substrate balance, and appetite profile', *Am J Clin Nutr* 2009; 89(3): 831–38

3. Halton, T L *et al.*, 'The Effects of High Protein Diets on Thermogenesis, Satiety and Weight Loss: A Critical Review', *J Am Coll of Nutr* 2004; 23(5): 373–85

4. Foster-Schubert, K E *et al.*, 'Acyl and total ghrelin are suppressed strongly by ingested proteins, weakly by lipids, and biphasically by carbohydrates', *J Clin Endocrinol Metab* 2008; 93(5): 1971–79

5. Weigle, D S *et al.*, 'A high-protein diet induces sustained reductions in appetite, ad libitum caloric intake, and body weight despite compensatory changes in diurnal

plasma leptin and ghrelin concentrations', *Am J Clin Nutr* 2005; 82(1): 41–48

6. Samaha, F F *et al.*, 'A low carbohydrate as compared with a low fat diet in severe obesity', *N Eng J Med* 2003; 348: 2074–81
7. Skov, A R *et al.*, 'Randomized trial on protein vs carbohydrate in ad libitum fat reduced diet for the treatment of obesity', *Int J Obes* 1999; 23: 528–36
8. Brehm, B J *et al.*, 'A randomized trial comparing a very low carbohydrate diet and a calorie restricted low fat diet on body weight and cardiovascular risk factors in healthy women', *J Clin Endocrinol Metab* 2003; 88: 1617–23
9. Yancy, W S Jr *et al.*, 'A low-carbohydrate, ketogenic diet versus a low-fat diet to treat obesity and hyperlipidemia', *Ann Intern Med* 2004; 140: 769–77
10. Skov, A R *et al.*, op cit
11. Walker Lasker, D A *et al.*, 'Moderate carbohydrate, moderate protein weight loss diet reduces cardiovascular disease risk compared to high carbohydrate, low protein diet in obese adults: A randomized clinical trial', *Nutrition & Metabolism* 2008; 5: 30
12. Brehm, B J *et al.*, op cit
13. Parker B *et al.*, 'Effect of a high protein, high monounsaturated fat weight loss diet on glycemic control and lipid levels in type-2 diabetes' *Diabetes Care* 2002; 25: 425–30
14. McAuley, K A *et al.*, 'Comparison of high-fat and high-protein diets with a high-carbohydrate diet in insulin-resistant obese women', *Diabetologia* 2005; 48(1): 8–16
15. Clifton, P M *et al.*, 'High protein diets decrease total and abdominal fat and improve CVD risk profile in overweight and obese men and women with elevated

triacylglycerol', *Nutr Metab Cardiovasc Dis* 2009; 19(8): 548–54

16. McAuley, K A *et al.*, 'Comparison of high-fat and high-protein diets with a high-carbohydrate diet in insulin-resistant obese women', *Diabetologia* 2005; 48(1): 8–16

17. Claessens, M *et al.*, 'The effect of a low-fat, high-protein or high-carbohydrate ad libitum diet on weight loss maintenance and metabolic risk factors', *Int J Obes (Lond)* 2009; 33(3): 296–304

18. Layman, D K *et al.*, 'A Moderate-Protein Diet Produces Sustained Weight Loss and Long-Term Changes in Body Composition and Blood Lipids in Obese Adults', *J Nutr* 2009; 139: 514–21

19. Krieger, J W *et al.*, 'Effects of variation in protein and carbohydrate intake on body mass and composition during energy restriction: a meta-regression 1', *Am J Clin Nutr* 2006; 83(2): 260–74

20. Layman, D K *et al.*, 'A reduced ratio of dietary carbohydrate to protein improves body composition and blood lipid profiles during weight loss in adult women' *J Nutr* 2003; 133(2): 411–17

21. Layman, D K *et al.*, 'Dietary protein and exercise have additive effects on body composition during weight loss in adult women', *J Nutr* 2005; 135(8): 1903–10

22. Nordestgaard, B G *et al.*, 'Non-fasting triglycerides and risk of myocardial infarction, ischemic heart disease, and death in men and women', *JAMA* 2007; 298(3): 299–308

23. Hu, F B, 'Protein, body weight, and cardiovascular health', *American Journal of Clinical Nutrition* 2005; 82(1); 242S–247S

24. Eisenstein, J *et al.*, 'High-protein weight loss diets: are they safe and do they work? A review of the

experimental and epidemiologic data', *Nutr Rev* 2002; 60: 189–200

25. Manninen, A H, 'High-protein weight loss diets and purported adverse effects: where is the evidence?', *Sports Nutrition Review Journal* 2004; 1(1): 45–51

26. Poortmans, J R *et al.*, 'Do regular high protein diets have potential health risks on kidney function in athletes?', *Int J Sport Nur Exerc Metab* 2000; 10: 28–38

27. Morgan, K T, 'Nutritional determinants of bone health', *J Nutr Elder* 2008; 27(1–2): 3–27

28. Conigrave, A D *et al.*, 'Dietary protein and bone health: roles of amino acid-sensing receptors in the control of calcium metabolism and bone homeostasis', *Annu Rev Nutr* 2008; 28: 131–55

29. Cordain, L *et al.*, 'Plant-animal subsistence ratios and macronutrient energy estimations in worldwide hunter-gatherer diets', *Am J Clin Nutr* 2000; 71(3): 682–92

CHAPTER 6

1. Beglinger, C *et al.*, 'Fat in the intestine as a regulator of appetite-role of CCK', *Physiol Behav* 2004; 83(4): 617–21

2. Melanson, K J *et al.*, 'Blood glucose patterns and appetite in time-blinded humans: carbohydrate versus fat', *Am J Physiol* 1999; 277(2 Pt 2): R337–45

3. Cecil, J E *et al.*, 'Comparison of the effects of a high-fat and high-carbohydrate soup delivered orally and intragastrically on gastric emptying, appetite, and eating behaviour', *Physiol Behav* 1999; 67(2): 299–306

4. Speechly, D P *et al.*, 'Acute appetite reduction associated with an increased frequency of eating in obese males', *International Journal of Obesity and Related Metabolic Disorders* 1999; 23(11): 1151–59

5. Jenkins, D J *et al.*, 'Nibbling versus gorging: advantages

of increased meal frequency', *N Engl J Med* 1989; 321(14): 929–34

6. Rashidi, M R, *et al.*, 'Effects of nibbling and gorging on lipid profiles, blood glucose and insulin levels in healthy subjects', *Saudi Med J* 2003; 24(9): 945–48

7. Farschi, R H *et al.*, 'Beneficial metabolic effects of regular meal frequency on dietary thermogenesis, insulin sensitivity, and fasting lipid profiles in healthy obese women', *Am J Clin Nutr* 2005; 81(1): 16–24

8. Ruidavets, J B *et al.*, 'Eating frequency and body fatness in middle-aged men', *Int J Obes Relat Metab Disord* 2002; 26(11): 1476–83

9. Fabry, P *et al.*, 'The frequency of meals: its relationship to overweight, hypercholesteremia, and decreased glucose-tolerance', *Lancet* 1964; 2: 614–15

10. Anton, S D *et al.*, 'Effects of chromium picolinate on food intake and satiety', *Diabetes Technol Ther* 2008; 10(5): 405–12

11. Docherty, J P *et al.*, 'A double-blind, placebo-controlled, exploratory trial of chromium picolinate in atypical depression: effect on carbohydrate craving', *J Psychiatr Pract* 2005; 11(5): 302–14

12. http://www.ku.dk/english/news/?content=http://www.ku.dk/english/news/dark_chokolate.htm

13. Fernandez-Tresguerres Hernández, J A, 'Effect of monosodium glutamate given orally on appetite control (a new theory for the obesity epidemic)', *An R Acad Nac Med* (Madr) 2005; 122(2): 341–55

14. Akira, Niijimab *et al.*, 'Cephalic-phase insulin release induced by taste stimulus of monosodium glutamate (umami taste)', *Physiology & Behavior* 1990; 48(6): 905–908

15. He, K *et al.*, 'Association of Monosodium Glutamate Intake with Overweight in Chinese Adults: The

INTERMAP Study', *Obesity* 2008; 16(8): 1875-80

16. Dolnikoff, M *et al.*, 'Decreased lipolysis and enhanced glycerol and glucose utilization by adipose tissue prior to development of obesity in monosodium glutamate (MSG) treated rats', *Int J Obes Relat Metab Disord* 2001; 25(3): 426-33

17. Frank, G K *et al.*, 'Sucrose activates human taste pathways differently from artificial sweetener', *Neuroimage* 2008; 39(4): 1559-69

18. Just, T *et al.*, 'Cephalic phase insulin release in healthy humans after taste stimulation?', *Appetite* 2008; 51(3): 622-27

19. Rogers, P J *et al.*, 'Separating the actions of sweetness and calories: effects of saccharin and carbohydrates on hunger and food intake in human subjects', *Physiol Behav* 1989; 45: 1093-99

20. Lavin, J H *et al.*, 'The Effect of Sucrose- and Aspartame-Sweetened Drinks on Energy Intake, Hunger and Food Choice of Female, Moderately Restrained Eaters', *International Journal of Obesity* 1997; 21: 37-42

21. Tordoff, M G *et al.*, 'Oral stimulation with aspartame increases hunger', *Physiol Behav* 1990; 47: 555-59

22. Swithers, S E *et al.*, 'A role for sweet taste: Calorie predictive relations in energy regulation by rats', *Behavioral Neuroscience* 2008; 122(1): 161-73

23. He, F J *et al.*, 'Salt intake is related to soft drink consumption in children and adolescents: a link to obesity?', *Hypertension* 2008; 51(3): 629-34

24. Maruyama, K *et al.*, 'The joint impact on being overweight of self reported behaviours of eating quickly and eating until full: cross sectional survey', *BMJ* 2008; 337: a2002

25. Study presented at the Annual meeting of the North American Association for the Study of Obesity. 20-

24 October 2006, Hynes Convention Center, Boston, Massachusetts, USA

26. Zijlstra, N *et al.*, 'Effect of bite size and oral processing time of a semisolid food on satiation', *Am J Clin Nutr* 2009; 90(2): 269-75

CHAPTER 7

1. Heizer, W D *et al.*, 'The role of diet in symptoms of irritable bowel syndrome in adults: a narrative review', *J Am Diet Assoc* 2009; 109(7): 1204-14

2. Jitomir, J *et al.*, 'Leucine for retention of lean mass on a hypocaloric diet', *J Med Food* 2008; 11(4): 606-609

3. Ponnampalam, E N *et al.*, 'Effect of feeding systems on omega-3 fatty acids, conjugated linoleic acid and trans fatty acids in Australian beef cuts: potential impact on human health', *Asia Pac J Clin Nutr* 2006; 15(1): 21-29

4. Engel, L S *et al.*, 'Population Attributable Risks of Esophageal and Gastric Cancers', *Journal of the National Cancer Institute* 2003; 95(18): 1404-13

5. Sarasua, S *et al.*, 'Cured and broiled meat consumption in relation to childhood cancer: Denver, Colorado (United States)', *Cancer Causes Control* 1994; 5(2): 141-48

6. Larsson, S C *et al.*, 'Meat consumption and risk of colorectal cancer: a meta-analysis of prospective studies', *Int J Cancer* 2006; 119(11): 2657-64

7. Truswell, A S, 'Meat consumption and cancer of the large bowel', *Eur J Clin Nutr* 2002; (Suppl 1): 19-24

8. Norat, T *et al.*, 'Meat consumption and colorectal cancer risk: dose–response meta-analysis of epidemiological studies', *Int J Cancer* 2002; 98(2): 241-56

9. Mozaffarian, D *et al.*, 'Fish Intake, Contaminants, and Human Health: Evaluating the Risks and the Benefits',

JAMA 2006; 296: 1885–99

10. Key, T J A *et al.*, 'Dietary habits and mortality in 11,000 vegetarians and health conscious people: results of a 17 year follow up', *BMJ* 1996; 313: 775–79

11. Thorogood, M *et al.*, 'Risk of death from cancer and ischemic heart disease in meat and non-meat eaters', *BMJ* 1994; 308: 1667–70

12. Key, T J *et al.*, 'Mortality in British vegetarians: results from the European Prospective Investigation into Cancer and Nutrition (EPIC-Oxford)', *Am J Clin Nutr* 2009; 89(5): 1613S–1619S

13. Mente, A *et al.*, 'A Systematic Review of the Evidence Supporting a Causal Link Between Dietary Factors and Coronary Heart Disease', *Arch Intern Med* 2009; 169(7): 659–69

14. Lajolo, F M *et al.*, 'Nutritional significance of lectins and enzyme inhibitors from legumes', *J Agric Food Chem* 2002; 50(22): 6592–6598

15. Darmadi-Blackberry, I *et al.*, 'Legumes: the most important dietary predictor of survival in older people of different ethnicities', *Asia Pac J Clin Nutr* 2004; 13(2): 217–20

16. Vidal-Valverde C *et al.*, 'Changes in the carbohydrate composition of legumes after soaking and cooking', *J Am Diet Assoc* 1993; 93(5): 547–50

17. El Tiney, A H, 'Proximate Composition and Mineral and Phytate Contents of Legumes Grown in Sudan', *Journal of Food Composition and Analysis* 1989; 2: 67–68

18. Rackis, J J *et al.*, 'The USDA trypsin inhibitor study. I. Background, objectives and procedural details', *Qualification of Plant Foods in Human Nutrition* 1985; 35

19. Rackis, J J, 'Biological and physiological Factors in Soybeans', *Journal of the American Oil Chemists'*

Society 1974; 51: 161–70

20. Divi, R L *et al.*, 'Anti-thyroid isoflavones from the soybean', *Biochemical Pharmacology* 1997; 54: 1087–96

21. Gikas, P D *et al.*, 'Phytoestrogens and the risk of breast cancer: a review of the literature', *Int J Fertil Women's Med* 2005; 50(6): 250–58

22. White, L, 'Association of High Midlife Tofu Consumption with Accelerated Brain Aging', Plenary Session 8: Cognitive Function, The Third International Soy Symposium, Program, November 1999; 26

23. Chavarro, J E *et al.*, 'Soy food and isoflavone intake in relation to semen quality parameters among men from an infertility clinic', *Hum Reprod* 2008; 23(11): 2584–90

24. Doerge, D R, 'Inactivation of Thyroid Peroxidase by Genistein and Daidzein in Vitro and in Vivo; Mechanism for Anti-Thyroid Activity of Soy', presented at the November 1999 Soy Symposium in Washington, DC, National Center for Toxicological Research, Jefferson, AR 72029, USA

25. http: //www.cspinet.org/new/200208121.html

26. http: //www.cspinet.org/quorn/

27. Hu, F B *et al.*, 'Frequent nut consumption and risk of coronary heart disease in women: prospective cohort study', *BMJ* 1998; 317(7169): 1341–45

28. Albert, C M *et al.*, 'Nut consumption and decreased risk of sudden cardiac death in the Physicians' Health Study', *Arch Intern Med* 2002; 162(12): 1382–87

29. Loones, A, 'Transformation of milk components during yogurt fermentation', in Chandan, R C (ed), *Yoghurt: nutritional and health properties* (McLean, VA: National Yoghurt Association, 1989): 95–114

30. Beshkova, D M *et al.*, 'Production of amino acids by

yoghurt bacteria', *Biotechnol Prog* 1998; 14: 963–65

CHAPTER 8

1. Chan, J *et al.*, 'Water, other fluids, and fatal coronary heart disease: the Adventist Health Study', *Am J Epidemiol* 2002; 155(9): 827–33

2. Wilkens, L R *et al.*, 'Risk factors for lower urinary tract cancer: the role of total fluid consumption, nitrites and nitrosamines, and selected foods', *Cancer Epidemiol Biomarkers Prev* 1996; 5: 116–66

3. Shannon, J *et al.*, 'Relationship of food groups and water intake to colon cancer risk', *Cancer Epidemiol Biomarkers Prev* 1996; 5: 495–502

4. Schliess, F *et al.*, 'Cell hydration and mTOR-dependent signalling', *Acta Physiol* (Oxford) 2006; 187: 223–29

5. Bilz, S *et al.*, 'Effects of hypoosmolality on whole-body lipolysis in man', *Metabolism* 1999; 48: 472–76

6. Keller, U *et al.*, 'Effects of changes in hydration on protein, glucose and lipid metabolism in man: impact on health', *Eur J Clin Nutr* 2003; 57(2): S69–S74

7. Armstrong, L E *et al.*, 'Urinary indices of hydration status', *Int J Sport Nutr* 1994; 4: 265–79

8. Gardner, E J *et al.*, 'Black tea – helpful or harmful? A review of the evidence', *Eur J Clin Nutr* 2006; 61: 3–18

9. Larsson, S C *et al.*, 'Coffee and Tea Consumption and Risk of Stroke Subtypes in Male Smokers', *Stroke* 2008; 39: 1681–87

10. Cabrera, C *et al.*, 'Beneficial effects of green tea – a review', *J Am Coll Nutr* 2006; 25(2): 79–99

11. Ibid.

12. Venables, M C *et al.*, 'Green tea extract ingestion, fat oxidation, and glucose tolerance in healthy humans', *Am J Clin Nutr* 2008; 87: 778–84

13. Boschmann, M *et al.*, 'The Effects of Epigallocatechin-3-Gallate on Thermogenesis and Fat Oxidation in Obese Men: A Pilot Study', *J Am Col Nutr* 2007; 26(4): 389S–395S
14. Nagao, T *et al.*, 'Ingestion of a tea rich in catechins leads to a reduction in body fat and malondialdehyde-modified LDL in men', *Am J Clin Nutr* 2005; 81(1): 122–29
15. Khokhar, S *et al.*, 'Total phenol, catechin, and caffeine contents of teas commonly consumed in the United Kingdom', *J Agric Food Chem* 2002; 50(3): 565–70
16. Maki, K C *et al.*, 'Green Tea Catechin Consumption Enhances Exercise-Induced Abdominal Fat Loss in Overweight and Obese Adults', *J Nutr* 2009 139: 264–70
17. Golden, E B *et al.*, 'Green tea polyphenols block the anti-cancer effects of bortezomib and other boronic acid-based proteasome inhibitors', *Blood* 2009; 113(23): 5927–37
18. Greenberg, J A *et al.*, 'Coffee, diabetes and weight control', *Am J Clin Nutr* 2006; 84: 682–93
19. Odegaard, A O *et al.*, 'Coffee, tea, and incident type 2 diabetes: the Singapore Chinese Health Study', *Am J Clin Nutr* 2008; 88(4): 979–85
20. Van Dam, R M *et al.*, 'Coffee consumption and risk of type 2 diabetes: a systematic review', *JAMA* 2005 Jul 6; 294(1): 97–104
21. Hino, A *et al.*, 'Habitual coffee but not green tea consumption is inversely associated with metabolic syndrome. An epidemiological study in a general Japanese population', *Diabetes Res Clin Pract* 2007; 76(3): 383–89
22. Larsson, op cit
23. Eskelinen, M H *et al.*, 'Midlife Coffee and Tea Drinking

and the Risk of Late-Life Dementia: A Population-Based CAIDE Study', *J Alzheimer's Dis* 2009; 16(1): 85–91

24. Barranco Quintana, J L *et al.*, 'Alzheimer's disease and coffee: a quantitative review', *Neurol Res* 2007; 29(1): 91–5

25. Arendash, G W *et al.*, 'Caffeine protects Alzheimer's mice against cognitive impairment and reduces brain beta-amyloid production', *Neuroscience* 2006; 142(4): 941–52

26. Malik, V S *et al.*, 'Intake of sugar-sweetened beverages and weight gain: a systematic review', *Am J Clin Nutr* 2006; 84: 274–88

27. Johnson, R K *et al.* 'Dietary sugars intake and cardiovascular health. A scientific statement from the American Heart Association', *Circulation* 24 August 2009 [epub before print]

28. Sanchez, A *et al.*, 'Role of Sugars in Human Neutrophilic Phagocytosis', *Am J Clin Nutr* 1973; 261: 1180–84

29. Bernstein, J *et al.*, 'Depression of Lymphocyte Transformation Following Oral Glucose Ingestion', *Am J Clin Nutr* 1997; 30: 613

30. Ringsdorf, W *et al.*, 'Sucrose, Neutrophilic Phagocytosis and Resistance to Disease', *Dental Survey* 1976; 52(12): 46–48

31. Couzy, F *et al.*, 'Nutritional Implications of the Interaction Minerals', *Progressive Food and Nutrition Science* 1933; 17: 65–87

32. Kozlovsky, A *et al.*, 'Effects of Diets High in Simple Sugars on Urinary Chromium Losses', *Metabolism* 1986; 35: 515–18

33. Fields, M *et al.*, 'Effect of Copper Deficiency on Metabolism and Mortality in Rats Fed Sucrose or Starch Diets', *Journal of Clinical Nutrition* 1983; 113: 1335–45

34. Lemann, J, 'Evidence that Glucose Ingestion Inhibits

Net Renal Tubular Reabsorption of Calcium and Magnesium', *Journal of Clinical Nutrition* 1976 ; 70: 236–45

35. Reiser, S *et al.*, 'Effects of Sugars on Indices on Glucose Tolerance in Humans', *Am J Clin Nutr* 1986; 43: 151–59

36. Le, K A *et al.*, 'A 4-week high fructose diet alters lipid metabolism without affecting insulin sensitivity or ectopic lipids in healthy humans', *Am J Clin Nutr* 2006; 84(6): 1374–79

37. Elliott, S S *et al.*, 'Fructose, weight gain and the insulin resistance syndrome', *Am J Clin Nutr* 2002; 76(5): 911–22

38. Johnson, R K *et al.*, op cit

39. Vartanian, LR *et al.*, 'Effects of soft drink consumption on nutrition and health: a systematic review and meta-analysis', *Am J Public Health* 2007; 97: 667–75

40. Soffritti, M *et al.*, 'First experimental demonstration of the multipotential carcinogenic effects of aspartame administered in the feed to Sprague–Dawley rats', *Environ Health Perspect* 2006; 114(3): 379–85

41. Van Den Eeden, S K *et al.*, ,Aspartame Ingestion and Headaches: A Randomized, Crossover Trial,' *Neurology* 1994; 44: 1787–1793

42. Lipton, R B *et al.*, 'Aspartame as a dietary trigger of headache.' *Headache* 1989; 29(2): 90–92

43. Walton, R G *et al.*, 'Adverse reactions to aspartame: double-blind challenge in patients from a vulnerable population,' *Biol Psychiatry* 1993; 34(1–2): 13–17

44. http: //www.dorway.com/peerrev.html

45. Bazzano, L A *et al.*, 'Intake of Fruit, Vegetables, and Fruit Juices and Risk of Diabetes in Women,' *Diabetes Care*, 2008; 31(7): 1311–7

46. Lukasiewicz, E *et al.*, 'Alcohol intake in relation to body mass index and waist-to-hip ratio: the importance of

type of alcoholic beverage,' *Public Health Nutr* 2005; 8(3): 315–20

47. Dallongeville, J *et al.*, 'Influence of alcohol consumption and various beverages on waist girth and waist-to-hip ratio in a sample of French men and women,' *Int J Obes Relat Metab Disord*. 1998; 22(12): 1178–83

48. Wannamethee, S G *et al.*, 'Alcohol and adiposity: effects of quantity and type of drink and time relation with meals,' *Int J Obes (Lond)*, 2005; 29(12): 1436–44

49. White, I R *et al.*, 'Alcohol consumption and mortality: modelling risks for men and women at different ages,' *BMJ*. 2002; 325: 191

50. McCann, S E *et al.*, 'Alcoholic beverage preference and characteristics of drinkers and nondrinkers in western New York (United States),' *Nutr Metab Cardiovasc Dis* 2003; 13(1): 2–11

51. Tjonneland, A M *et al.*, 'The connection between food and alcohol intake habits among 48, 763 Danish men and women. A cross-sectional study in the project "Food, cancer and health",' *Ugeskr Laeger*. 1999; 161(50): 6923–7

52. Barefoot, J C *et al.*, 'Alcohol beverage preference, diet and health habits in the UNC Alumni Heart Study,' *Am J Clin Nutr* 2002; 76(2): 466–72

CHAPTER 10

1. Boden, G *et al.*, 'Effect of a low-carbohydrate diet on appetite, blood glucose levels, and insulin resistance in obese patients with type 2 diabetes', *Ann Intern Med* 2005; 142(6): 403–11

2. Melanson, E L *et al.*, 'Exercise improves fat metabolism in muscle but does not increase 24-h fat oxidation', *Exerc Sport Sci Rev* 2009; 37(2): 93–101

3. Finlayson, G *et al.*, 'Acute compensatory eating

following exercise is associated with implicit hedonic wanting for food', *Physiol Behav* 2009; 97(1): 62–67

4. Shaw, K *et al.*, 'Exercise for overweight or obesity', *Cochrane Database of Systematic Reviews* 2006, Issue 4. Art. No.: CD003817

5. Fogelholm, M *et al.*, 'Does physical activity prevent weight gain – a systematic review', *Obes Rev* 2000; 1(2): 95–111

6. Catenacci, V A *et al.*, 'The role of physical activity in producing and maintaining weight loss', *Nat Clin Pract Endocrinol Metab* 2007; 3(7): 518–29

7. Tully, M A *et al.*, 'Randomised controlled trial of home-based walking programmes at and below current recommended levels of exercise in sedentary adults', *J Epidemiol Community Health* 2007; 61(9): 778–83

8. Andersen, L B, 'Physical activity and health. Even low intensity exercise such as walking is associated with better health', *BMJ* 2007; 334: 1173

9. Manson, J E *et al.*, 'A prospective study of walking as compared with vigorous exercise in the prevention of coronary heart disease in women', *N Engl J Med* 1999; 341: 650–58

10. Hu, F B *et al.*, 'Walking compared with vigorous physical activity and risk of type 2 diabetes in women', *JAMA* 1999; 282: 1433–39

11. Cannell, J J *et al.*, 'Athletic Performance and Vitamin D', *Med Sci Sports Exerc* 2009; 41(5): 1102–10

12. Miyashita, M *et al.*, 'Accumulating short bouts of brisk walking reduces postprandial plasma triacylglycerol concentrations and resting blood pressure in healthy young men', *Am J Clin Nutr* 2008; 88(5): 1225–31

13. Schmidt, W D *et al.*, 'Effects of long versus short bout exercise on fitness and weight loss in overweight females', *J Am Coll Nutr* 2001; 20(5): 494–501

14. Bravata, D M *et al.*, 'Using pedometers to increase physical activity and improve health: a systematic review', *JAMA* 2007; 298(19): 2296–2304
15. Geliebter, A *et al.*, 'Effects of strength or aerobic training on body composition, resting metabolic rate, and peak oxygen consumption in obese dieting subjects', *Am J Clin Nutr* 1997; 66(3): 557–63
16. Stiegler, P *et al.*, 'The role of diet and exercise for the maintenance of fat-free mass and resting metabolic rate during weight loss', *Sports Med* 2006; 36(3): 239–62
17. Ruiz, J R *et al.*, 'Association between muscular strength and mortality in men: prospective cohort study', *BMJ* 2008; 337: a439
18. Phinney, S D, 'Ketogenic diets and physical performance', *Nutr Metab* (Lond) 2004; 1: 2

CHAPTER 11

1. Crum, A J *et al.*, 'Mind-set matters: exercise and the placebo effect', *Psychol Sci* 2007; 18(2): 165–71
2. Framson, C *et al.*, 'Development and validation of the mindful eating questionnaire', *J Am Diet Assoc* 2009; 109(8): 1439–44
3. Ranganathan, V K *et al.*, 'From mental power to muscle power – gaining strength by using the mind', *Neuropsychologia* 2004; 42(7): 944–56
4. Yue, G *et al.*, 'Strength increases from the motor program: comparison of training with maximal voluntary and imagined muscle contractions', *J Neurophysiol* 1992; 67(5): 1114–23
5. Zijdewind, I *et al.*, 'Effects of imagery motor training on torque production of ankle plantar flexor muscles', *Muscle Nerve* 2003; 28(2): 168–73

ACKNOWLEDGMENTS

To Robert Kirby, my agent, and Michelle Pilley, managing director of Hay House, UK – both of whom are always an absolute pleasure and inspiration to work with.

To the whole Hay House team, including Jo Burgess, Simon Gaske, Jessica Crockett and Duncan Carson – for their hard work, efficiency and good humour.

To Joe Briffa, Dr Peter Robbins and Greg Mead – for their invaluable comments on early drafts of this book.

To Chris Williams, Chris Swain, Charlie Cannon and Matt Blakely – for their help and advice regarding the exercise routine in chapter 10.

To Jyotish Patel, John Bennett and Sera Irvine – for the culinary know-how and creativity which went into many of the recipes in this book.

To Sandra Gomes and Jo Orchard – for their suggestions and expertise regarding the final chapter.

To Barbara Vesey, my editor – for being so efficient and easy to work with.

To a great number of individuals who I have met professionally and have somehow inspired or supported my work (and many of whom have turned into good friends!) including David Adams, Jean-Marc Barbeau, Janice Barry, Steve Boley, Andi Britt, Austin Caffrey, Lianne Campbell, Sarah Clarke, David Coleman, Nicky Cooling, Paul Davies, Dr Albert Ferrante, Dr Nicola Hembry, Tim Kyndt, Michelle Loughney, Keith Mansfield, Emma Markwick, Wayne McFarlane, Dr Ron Miller, Dr Bill Mitchell, Elena Petevi, Ian Powell, David Prosser, Dr Bernard Shevlin, Rebecca Stevens, Roger Thomas, Deborah Vandepeer, Dick Watkin, Garry Watts and Paul Woolston.

To my parents Dr Joseph Briffa and Dr Dorothy Burgess – for their enduring love, support and encouragement.

And last, but most certainly not least, to Sandra Gomes – for the countless blessings she has bestowed on me, that I am eternally grateful for.

ABOUT THE AUTHOR

Dr John Briffa BSc (Hons) MB BS

Dr John Briffa is a practising doctor, author and international speaker. He is a prize-winning graduate of University College London School of Medicine, where he also gained a BSc degree in Biomedical Sciences. Dr Briffa is a leading authority on the impact of nutrition and other lifestyle factors on health and illness. In his work, he is dedicated to providing individuals with information and advice they can use to take control of their health and optimise their energy and vitality.

Dr Briffa is a former columnist for the *Daily Mail* and the *Observer*, and former contributing editor for *Men's Health* magazine. He has contributed to over 100 newspaper and magazine titles internationally, and is a previous recipient of the Health Journalist of the Year award in the UK. He has been listed by Tatler magazine as one of the UK's leading doctors, and has twice been on the judging panel of the prestigious Prince of Wales Integrated Health Awards. *Waist Disposal* is Dr Briffa's seventh book.

In addition to his work in clinical practice and writing, for the last 15 years Dr Briffa has regularly delivered talks, workshops and courses geared towards the optimisation of energy, effectiveness and sustainability in individuals within organisations. Corporate clients include PricewaterhouseCoopers, Reuters, IBM, Bank of England, Morgan Stanley, Baker and Mackenzie, Bovis Lendlease, Danone, Deloitte, Clifford Chance, Eversheds, GE Money, GE Capital, Skandia, SSL International and BP.

Dr Briffa also offers nutritional consulting services to the business world, including an online nutrition profiling tool (Nutrinalysis™). This unique product provides an individualised report encompassing dietary analysis, as well as specific, tailored recommendations on dietary changes for optimal energy, wellbeing and general health. See **www.nutrinalysis.net** for more details.

For more details regarding Dr John Briffa and his work see **www.drbriffa.com**

CONTACT DETAILS:

Dr John Briffa can be contacted at:

Woolaston House
17-19 View Road
Highgate
London
N6 4DJ
UK

Tel: +44 (0) 208 341 3422
Fax: +44 (0) 208 340 1376

Email: john@drbriffa.com

For more information on Dr John Briffa's products and services (including workshops, e-books, podcasts and other electronic educational products), to read his regularly updated blog, and to sign up for his *free* weekly e-newsletter, go to **www.drbriffa.com**

INDEX

JOIN THE HAY HOUSE FAMILY

As the leading self-help, mind, body and spirit publisher in the UK, we'd like to welcome you to our family so that you can enjoy all the benefits our website has to offer.

 EXTRACTS from a selection of your favourite author titles

 COMPETITIONS, PRIZES & SPECIAL OFFERS Win extracts, money off, downloads and so much more

 LISTEN to a range of radio interviews and our latest audio publications

 CELEBRATE YOUR BIRTHDAY An inspiring gift will be sent your way

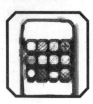 **LATEST NEWS** Keep up with the latest news from and about our authors

 ATTEND OUR AUTHOR EVENTS Be the first to hear about our author events

 iPHONE APPS Download your favourite app for your iPhone

 HAY HOUSE INFORMATION Ask us anything, all enquiries answered

join us online at **www.hayhouse.co.uk**

 292B Kensal Road, London W10 5BE
T: 020 8962 1230 E: info@hayhouse.co.uk